ART SMITH'S HEALTHY COMFORT

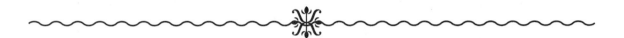

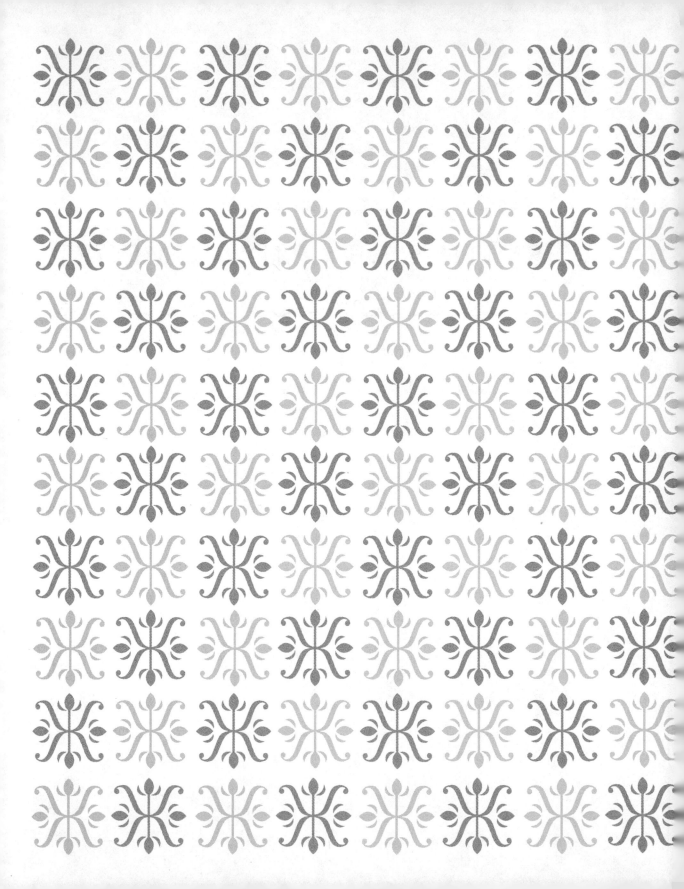

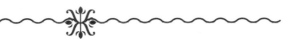

Art Smith's

HEALTHY
COMFORT

How America's Favorite Celebrity Chef

Got It Together, Lost Weight, and

Reclaimed His Health!

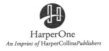

HarperOne
An Imprint of HarperCollinsPublishers

HarperOne

This book is written as a source of information only. The information contained in this book should by no means be considered a substitute for the advice of a qualified medical professional, who should always be consulted before beginning any new diet, exercise, or other health program.

HarperCollins books may be purchased for educational, business, or sales promotional use. For information, please e-mail the Special Markets Department at SPsales@harper collins.com.

HarperCollins website: http://www.harpercollins.com

HarperCollins®, 📖®, and HarperOne™ are trademarks of HarperCollins Publishers

FIRST EDITION

Photography by Stephen Hamilton
Designed by Jessica Shatan Heslin/Studio Shatan, Inc.

Library of Congress Cataloging-in-Publication Data
Smith, Art.
    Art Smith's healthy comfort : how America's favorite celebrity chef got it together, lost weight, and reclaimed his health! / by Art Smith. — First edition.
        pages cm
    Includes index.
    ISBN 978–0–06–221777–6
    1. Smith, Art. 2. Reducing diets—Recipes. 3. Overweight men—United States—Biography. 4. Celebrity chefs—Health and hygiene—United States. I. Title. II. Title: Healthy comfort.
    RM222.2.S616   2013
    613.2'5092—dc23
    [B]   2013000266

13 14 15 16 17 RRD(H) 10 9 8 7 6 5 4 3 2 1

For my late grandfather, Gilbert Arthur Jones,

and

For my late father, Palmer Gene Smith

CONTENTS

〜〜〜〜〜〜〜〜〜〜〜〜〜〜〜〜〜

Introduction ix

1 ❄ You Can Reclaim Your Health, Too! 1

2 ❄ How I Took the Plunge 9

3 ❄ Breakfast: Start the Day Right! 13

4 ❄ First Courses and Snacks 31

5 ❄ Soups 49

6 ❄ Salads 67

7 ❄ Vegetarian Main Courses 91

8 ❄ Fish and Seafood Main Courses 115

9 ❄ Meat and Poultry Main Courses 145

10 ❄ Vegetable Side Dishes 173

11 ❄ Party Day Foods: Treats Big and Small 197

A Note to My Readers 237

Acknowledgments 239

Index 243

INTRODUCTION

I f you've picked up this book, congratulations! You might be battling
with your weight, or perhaps you don't feel your best and want to
eat more healthfully. Maybe you are interested in good, wholesome
recipes for your family. Whatever the motivation, you're taking the
first step! That's great—and I know from experience that the first one
is the toughest. I hope my story and what I have learned will inspire
you to take charge of your life. You will be able to drop pounds, regain
your health, and learn to love the time spent in the kitchen preparing
one great-tasting *and* good-for-you dish after another.

Before I go any further, I want to be clear: this is not a "diet book"
in the classic sense. I make no claims that the recipes on these pages
will help you lose any specific number of pounds. Instead, they are full
of healthful, whole foods and great flavors that work with a healthy
lifestyle. The advice in this book is my own, too, and by following it, I
have turned my life around. Perhaps you can, too!

In the past several years, I have lost 120 pounds, wrestled type 2
diabetes into submission (or at least remission!), and become reacquainted with all sorts of foods in their most natural, whole state. I
cook in my beautiful home kitchen far more often than I used to because I realize how important it is to know exactly what I put in my
body.

But, Sweetie, let me tell you: it wasn't easy! And still isn't.

Back in the day, before my life changed for the better, food tasted
the most delicious when I felt the worst inside. Sound familiar? To the
world, I am outgoing, fun loving, and flirty. Since my school days in

North Florida I have loved an audience, and when I grew up I found a way to direct my skill as a chef into "celebrity" status so that I could perform as much as I pleased.

Yet below the surface of this jolly façade was a lot of self-hatred and doubt. Like so many people, I ate to combat the negativity and to fill a void. I was around food all day long, so this wasn't too hard, and no one seemed to notice when I packed on the pounds. I was a fat, jovial chef who cooked good-ole-boy southern food that the world loved.

Where It Began

I didn't realize how depressed I was when I tipped the scales at 325 pounds, but my health coach, Aaron (Az) Ferguson, recognized it from day one, as I describe in chapter 2, "How I Took the Plunge." His solution wasn't to send me to a psychiatrist but to get me walking, biking, and eating right. That's his job, and he knows what he's doing. He made me sweat, made me curb my out-of-control appetite, and taught me the value of a healthful lifestyle. He also assured me that everyone, fit or not, has issues to confront.

Issues? Did I say issues? You bet I had issues!

Where to begin? Childhood is as good a place as any, and mine was both idyllic and distressing. Living in a small southern town and knowing I was different was rough. I was gay and never quite fit in. When I was little, I found refuge in my mother's and grandmother's kitchens, hanging out with them and my wonderful aunts and cousins, all of whom were spectacular cooks. Some of my fondest memories are of family gatherings along the Suwannee River, where the deep springs created swimming holes that kept us kids enthralled for hours on end. If we were lucky, we might spot a gentle manatee swimming upstream from the Gulf of Mexico. After working up an appetite in the river, we'd gather along its banks to eat potato salad, deviled eggs, sweet potato pie, fried chicken, and coconut cake.

As I entered my teens, I decided I was adopted. My red hair stood out. I was completely different from my brother, who wanted to farm like our father did, while I wanted nothing to do with it. Instead I grabbed every opportunity to play the piano or perform on stage. Not surprisingly, I was bullied at school, although the misery it created was somewhat assuaged by the food my mother cooked. Later, as a young chef, I got a job at the Greenbrier, a large and prestigious resort in West Virginia. The older chefs bullied me mercilessly, so I escaped to the pastry kitchen, where the kindly pastry chef, Mark Gray, who taught me to make chocolate, which helped to ease the pain. To this day, I think of chocolate when I am upset.

Moving Forward

It might have been my determination to live life in a bigger world or it might have been the wretchedness that came with being so out of step with everyone around me that propelled me into the life I now have. Whatever it was, I have been blessed. Early on, I landed a job as the chef for Florida governor Bob Graham and later moved to Chicago, where I became a personal chef and caterer. I met a guy named Andre Walker, a hairdresser by trade who liked my cooking so much he mentioned me to his most famous client, Oprah Winfrey. I cooked for Ms. Winfrey (as I always called her, being a southern gentleman) for ten years. These days, I am on call for the many special events she hosts across the country. I learned so much from her about love, acceptance, and fellowship that I wouldn't know where to start if asked to define her most indispensable lesson.

Life was good. I wrote *Back to the Table,* which was a bestseller, and I also won a James Beard Award. I appeared frequently on Oprah's television show and discovered how much I liked being in front of the camera. I landed guest shots on food shows such as *Iron Chef; Extreme Makeover: Home Edition;* and later *Top Chef* and *Top Chef Masters.* I became a sought-after speaker and chef at all sorts of events across the nation. With Jesus Salgueiro, I founded Common Threads in 2003, a not-for-profit with a mission to teach low-income children about healthful eating and cooking.

Jesus and I also found love. Working with Oprah and others who accepted my sexuality made this easier than it would have been otherwise, but as anyone who has been in love knows, it wasn't a smooth road. We had our bumps! Combine the exigencies of romance with the stresses of a high-profile job and then add my embedded insecurities, and it's no surprise my weight ballooned. It took me a long time to realize I had always turned to food to alleviate stress and ease pain.

As my weight increased, medical experts on Oprah's show urged me to lose it. Both Dr. Mehmet Oz and Dr. Dean Ornish, two men who have influenced countless viewers and followers over the years, encouraged me to get a handle on my health. Jesus, who has been my partner for thirteen years, got sick in 2003; for the next four years, he battled cancer. I battled it right along with him and, not surprisingly, gained even more weight. Caregivers are vulnerable to this very real problem, and Jesus's doctor, Jeffrey Raizer, warned me to take care of myself. Three doctors told me to lose weight, and I didn't listen! Talk about denial.

When I finally decided to pay attention, I got help. That help took the form of Aaron (Az) Ferguson, a 24/7 health coach who, as I talk about throughout the book and particularly in chapter 2, "How I Took the Plunge," made all the difference for me. I know most people won't have the luxury of working with their own coach, but since I needed a lot of babysitting, I took full advantage of all Az had to offer. Years before, Az had overcome chronic back pain with exercise while waiting for Australia's health system to schedule an operation for him. That event persuaded him to become a professional coach, and to this day he takes on physical challenges as a way to elevate his own life.

Az advises those who want to become healthier to seek out the fittest, most health-conscious people they know. Talk to them, find out what they do, and gauge their attitude. Could you model some of your behavior after your chosen role model? Can he or she give you some tips for achieving success?

You're about to make big changes in your life. I'm behind you all the way. Find others who will take you seriously and be supportive. Believe it or not, some of your closest friends may not be among these folks. Some people are afraid of change, and if you decide to modify how you live and how you approach eating and exercise, it could threaten them. Get rid of these people, at least at the beginning of your efforts, or avoid social situations that include them. These may be the same friends who encourage you to split a large order of fries and a hot fudge sundae when you go out. You know who they are, or you will discover them as soon as you begin to change your habits.

You have to take care of you and you alone during this time. Your health is more important than anything else. If you aren't feeling your best or can't do things because your breath is labored and your knees hurt, you won't be much help to your loved ones. Try not to let anyone sabotage your decision to regain your health. Once your body is in top working order, your life will be easier to manage, you will feel a fantastic sense of accomplishment—and you will be full of joy.

ART SMITH'S HEALTHY COMFORT

You Can Reclaim Your Health, Too!

Why did I do it? What was the tipping point when I decided enough was enough and I wasn't going to put up with it anymore? I wish I could point to a single "eureka moment," but just as the extra hundred-plus pounds crept slowly onto my body, so the decision to shed them evolved over time.

There were moments along the way. I winced when I saw myself on TV, I struggled to find clothes that fit, and I wasn't comfortable sitting on planes, but like so many overweight people, I rationalized these away. I could live with these mere annoyances, right?

As do most people who know they are in trouble and should do something about it, I told myself again and again that I was still living the life I had carved out for myself and was doing just fine. My weight was not a hindrance to my success; at the time, I was a partner in two restaurants and a celebrity contestant on *Top Chef Masters* and other television programs. The phone kept ringing with people wanting me to do this and do that, so how could there possibly be a problem? And yet, in the back of my mind I knew I needed to lose weight. I couldn't bend down to tie my shoelaces . . . but even that red flag was shrugged off with slip-on shoes!

Diabetes and Me

Looking back, if there was one moment that convinced me to take charge, it was when I was diagnosed with type 2 diabetes. My father battled diabetes for years and eventually died from complications of the disease, so when in 2008 the doctor told me I, too, was afflicted, I freaked out.

I wish I could tell you that I left the doctor's office with a resolve of steel to lose weight and change my diet. Sure, I told myself I was going to get it under control, but I also spent a lot of time worrying and arguing with myself about its impact. My blood glucose levels were high enough that the doc put me on medication. Okay, I thought, one pill a day and I will be okay. I'll do a little something to rein in my voracious sweet tooth, and everything will fall into place.

But I am human and, as I said, my dad suffered from diabetes, so I did what any normal person would do: I panicked. I found myself waking up in the middle of the night, sweating and gasping for breath. I had bouts of insomnia—I feared falling asleep, thinking I might never wake up again. My blood pressure zipped up and down. I even rushed to the hospital a few times with "heart attacks," which actually were panic attacks. My mood swings were startling, especially since I am normally an outgoing, gregarious person not given to bouts of sadness and depression.

Unlike type 1 diabetes (which used to be called juvenile diabetes and must be controlled with insulin), type 2, my kind, often is manageable through diet and exercise. It's also the type of diabetes that afflicts the most people, by far. According to the American Diabetes Association, 25.8 million Americans have type 2 diabetes, and another 79 million, considered prediabetic, are in danger of developing it. In 2010 alone, 1.9 million of our fellow citizens were diagnosed with type 2 diabetes. The statistics are alarming—particularly as they reflect to some extent our unhealthy lifestyle. Too many Americans are obese and sedentary, two factors that very often contribute to type 2 diabetes.

When I came to terms with what could happen if I didn't "own" the disease, I was more than a little anxious. People with out-of-control type 2 diabetes have significantly higher incidences of high blood pressure, heart disease and stroke, kidney disease, blindness, neuropathy, and amputations. No, thank you!

I was frightened. The time had come to take charge.

In the end, I count myself among the lucky ones because once I got my act together, I was able to control my disease with diet and exercise. Oprah even devoted a television show to my triumph as a message to other diabetics. Many, if not most, type 2 diabetics can do the same. You still must be vigilant about monitoring glucose levels and seeing the doctor regularly, but you can manage diabetes and live a healthy, active, and long life.

Reclaim Your Health!

Most people reading this book don't have type 2 diabetes, but a lot of you are struggling with extra weight. If you are heavy, you may also be in failing health, or will be at a later date if you don't do something about it now.

Let's see. I checked with the Centers for Disease Control, which confirmed what most of us know. Obesity is a contributor to coronary heart disease, stroke, hypertension, high cholesterol and triglycerides, liver and gallbladder disease, osteoarthritis, some cancers (including endometrial, breast, and colon), sleep apnea, and respiratory problems; it can even affect fertility in women. And, of course, it can cause type 2 diabetes.

I got my health back by working very hard for nearly three years to lose 120 pounds—and keep it off. In the next chapter, I go into more detail about how my coach, Az Ferguson, guided me through the process. I realize most people don't have a personal health coach, so I decided to write a book that details my journey to help others find their own path.

It's not easy. God knows I fell off the wagon time and time again. But I got into the habit of waking up the next day more determined than ever to push forward. I ate right, learned a lot about food that even I, a trained chef, didn't know, and came to value exercise as part of my day. I hope this book will help you reclaim your good health, or hold on to it. As I point out in the introduction, this is not a diet book. The recipes included here are not meant to help you dramatically drop pounds as much as they are reminders of how to eat right, healthfully, and sensibly, day in and day out, without any sacrifice of flavor, satisfaction, or the joy of gathering around the table with those you love.

Good Food, Bad Food

Time was when I didn't believe any food was "bad," and overall I still don't. What is bad is how we treat the wonderful bounty found on our planet. We tend to cook with a lot of fat and sugar, to transform perfectly honest food so that it becomes a risk to our health. Think about a good-size beef hamburger topped with cheese and bacon. As the saying goes, it's a heart attack on a plate. Now, there is nothing intrinsically wrong with beef, cheese, or bacon eaten separately and in moderation. All are high in fat, but they also are good sources of protein. None is considered a "health food," but that does not mean you have to give them up, and the same is true for any number of tasty foods.

Instead of worrying about "giving up" certain foods, it's far more fun and liberating to think about those foods you should embrace when you decide to take control of your health. The most important word in my new, updated and powerful vocabulary is *whole*. Try to eat foods as close to their whole and most natural states as you can. This means an apple instead of apple pie, steamed green beans and pea pods instead of the same doused with melted cheese, and a perfectly browned roasted chicken rather than a chicken and noodle casserole or fried chicken.

When you eat a fresh nectarine, bursting with juiciness from the summer sun, or a fish recently caught from a nearby body of water, you can almost taste the health. These foods have not been adulterated, stored for too long, or treated with chemicals or additives to prolong their shelf life.

I'm an omnivore. I eat just about everything, including meat, and I enjoy every bite. This does not mean I don't look forward to meals that are mostly vegetarian or even vegan, because I do. I have a chapter dedicated to vegetarian main courses, and I am very happy with every recipe. When I was deciding on what dishes to include in the chapter on vegetable side dishes, I had a terrible time winnowing it down to a manageable number. I have come to love, love, love vegetables in the past few years and have dreamed up countless ways to prepare them, many of which I share with you in these recipes. I always appreciated vegetables, but now I think of them as the king of the food chain.

If vegetables are the king, fruit has to be the queen—sweet, tempting, and satisfying. Although you can't eat fruit with the same abandon as vegetables, you can eat it happily and without guilt. It's a wonderful dessert and a tasty snack. No one ever got fat from eating too many clementines! Fruit is packed with natural sugars and, like veggies, valuable vitamins and necessary fiber. There really is not much to complain about with them either, except perhaps when you buy them out of season and are rewarded with a mealy apple or a tasteless asparagus spear.

I am not going to continue the metaphor (cheese as the knave of the food world, whole grains as the princes?), but I want to emphasize what you *should* eat every day. It's far more fun to decide what to eat than to worry about what not to eat.

As you may know, I start nearly every day with oatmeal mixed with fruit and thick Greek yogurt. I explain why in more detail in the introduction to the breakfast chapter on page 13 and in the sidebar titled "Opting for Oatmeal" on page 17. I try to eat a simple protein, such as a chicken breast, lean steak, or ground turkey for lunch, accompanied by a salad or vegetable side dish. When dinner rolls around, I eat lightly if I am at home; if I am out, I stick with preparations that are as close as possible to the whole food. This means I avoid heavy sauces and fussy garnishes and instead choose grilled salmon (one of my favorites) or pan-seared lamb chops or chicken breast. Sometimes I just order two appetizers and delight in their heady flavors and small portions. I choose whole grains and legumes whenever possible. Grain salads and dishes based on beans not only taste great but are full of fiber and crucial nutrients.

I am a big fan of salads. I know, I know. Salads aren't manly, but let me tell you, a big green salad every day will keep your innards running as smoothly as clockwork! And they taste good, too. I steer clear of too much cheese, greedy handfuls of croutons, or heavy creamy dressings and instead go for nicely seasoned vinaigrettes (or dressings, as we call them in the South) that can be served on the side. If you taste all the different lettuces out there, from buttery Bibb to crisp romaine and peppery arugula, you won't want to obscure them with gobs of dressing. And speaking of salad dressing, it's never a bad investment to buy the best, fruitiest extra-virgin olive oil you can afford and pair it with a high-quality vinegar. The former is a terrific source of monounsaturated fat and amazing flavor, and the latter is calorie-free and the perfect pick-me-up for so many dishes.

Fat and Sugar

These are the culprits. These are what makes us fat and lazy. But oh, Honey! They taste so good! The truth is everyone needs some fat for energy and essential fatty acids to deliver fat-soluble vitamins to our bodies. Fat also is good for our skin. But before you get carried away and run out for a pint of chocolate chip mint, keep in mind that no one should get more than 35 percent of their calories from fat—and if you are trying to take off pounds and keep them off, it's a good idea to reduce that to 20 or 25 percent. Problem is, many of us consume up to 40 percent of our calories as fat.

When I eat fat, I pay attention to what kind of fat it is. "Good" fats are those that are monounsaturated and polyunsaturated, such as olive, canola, soy, corn, nut, and sunflower oils. These beneficial fats are present in peanut butter, avocados, fish, seeds, and nuts. What you want to avoid are saturated fats from red meat and dairy, especially full-fat dairy. Particularly dangerous are trans fats, which are found in processed foods and come from partially hydrogenated oil. Yes. Read the label when you buy anything you aren't sure of.

Refined sugar is a bigger problem than fat. Since I started investing in living healthfully, I have come to the realization that refined sugar is one nasty villain. I'm not talking here about the natural sugars that are found in fruits and vegetables, folks. No one wants to give up sugar and it's near impossible to do so, but I urge you to try. Cut back on sugary foods that are made with refined sugar, such as cereals, breads, cookies, soda, juice, and alcohol, and try to get your sweet fix from fruit and caramelized veggies. Read the sidebar on page 214 called "Sugar Ain't So Sweet" to get a good grasp on how insidious it is.

Refined sugar is a carbohydrate, and when it enters our bodies, it's digested quickly and rushes directly to our bloodstreams, causing insulin levels to spike and then plummet, which makes us hungry for more refined sugar. This is not good for our bodies, and over time it can cause some serious health issues, namely heart disease and diabetes. All this time, you have probably been more worried about getting heart disease from a T-bone steak and a sour-cream-topped baked potato, when perhaps you should be equally concerned with the sugary donut you munch every morning.

Exercise Makes a Difference

A lot of overweight, unhealthy people don't want to hear about exercise. They would rather sit on the couch eating raw carrots and sipping unsweetened iced tea than get up and move. The carrots and tea will help them drop the weight, right? And they can stay home and not face the world, not admit they have a problem.

Az taught me that it was okay to admit to my problems. No one wants to do it, he said, but once you "own" your weight gain, your failing health, your creaky joints and too-tight jeans, you can start to do something about them. Without 100 percent responsibility, you'll never regain your health and your body—and if you decide to take the victim route, forget it! Talk about negativity. Luckily, I am naturally open and gregarious. I was happy to unburden myself to Az and to any of my family and friends who would listen. When I got into exercise, I quickly realized how much time food had taken in my "other life." As a chef and restaurateur, I have to think about food; it's my livelihood. But I was also a big eater. I used to think about lunch when I was eating breakfast. I learned to channel my energy, as well as my stress and anxiety, into things other than food. I learned to breathe, to sit still for a few minutes, and also to relish the effects of working out. After a good run or an hour at the gym, I felt calm, strong, and energized all at once. I connected with the fact that my blood was flowing freely, my heart was strengthening, and my body was releasing good-for-me endorphins.

Finally, I realized that when you are in a good place, when your stress levels are under control, when you have decided to take charge of your well-being, you don't have to rely on food to help you feel better. You already are better.

A Word About Salt and Sodium

Finally, watch your sodium intake. In the nutritional facts following every recipe, I mention the amount of sodium. Some counts appear quite low, but read the recipe carefully. If I instruct you to add salt or to season "to taste," the amount can't be calculated in the sodium count. So, to err on the side of caution, sprinkle salt sparingly on the food when given the option to add it to suit your own taste. ❋

2

How I Took the Plunge

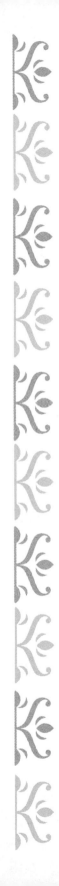

When I decided to lose weight, my guardian angel was watching over me: she took the form of Lisa Shotland, who was responsible for sending Az to my front door. I had been working the phones, trying to find the right person to help me shed a good number of my staggering 325 pounds, when I got a call from a stranger with a charming Aussie accent. It was Aaron (Az) Ferguson, recommended by Lisa, who assured me he could help. A week later, he was on my Chicago doorstep, having flown in from Los Angeles. He had his bags with him and moved right into our house! That way he could observe exactly what I ate and when I ate it. He could also figure out how much I exercised (not much in those days!).

Art, Az asked, what do you like to do for exercise? I told him I liked to walk, ride my bike, and dance. He smiled broadly. Well, he said, get ready to walk a lot, ride your bike a lot, and dance a lot! He wasn't kidding.

In the end, I discovered I also liked to run. Az says a lot of heavy folks turn out to be good runners because their legs are strong from carrying around so much weight. I never dreamed that would be me, but before too long our walks turned into jogs and the jogs into runs. As I describe on page 56 in the piece called "I've Run Marathons. Who Would Have Guessed?" I ran both the Chicago Marathon and the Marine Corps Marathon in the space of three weeks—with a lot of wonderful friends and fans cheering me on as I pounded along those mean city streets!

A New Way with Food

Soon after he arrived, Az set up a strict eating routine for me to follow. As he explained, most weight-loss diets are not healthy because they aren't balanced. By cutting back on calories, you often deprive the body of nutrients. While he believes that calorie reduction combined with exercise is the only way to lose weight, it's the calories you choose to omit that make a difference. It's important to have a specific plan and stick to it. The plan he put me on included good, wholesome foods, plenty of rest, and a lot of exercise.

I started each day with a bowl of oatmeal mixed with an egg white and berries. I still eat a variation of that breakfast every morning, but as you will read many times in this book, I now rely on thick, rich lowfat or nonfat Greek yogurt for protein and only sometimes add an egg white for an extra burst of protein. I ate a simple protein, such as chicken or fish, with a salad or steamed vegetable for both lunch and dinner, eating dinner early in the evening. Az quickly purged our kitchen of processed sugar, flour, white rice, and anything else that was not pure and true to his mission to get me on the straight and narrow when it came to my health, my weight, and my overall well-being.

He got me in the habit of drinking water. Before he entered my life, I was barely drinking any; instead I was downing a six-pack of Diet Coke every day. I am not sure of the science, but increasing the amount of water I drink and getting rid of the diet soda aided my weight loss and is a habit I happily continue. By the way, he tried to get me to forgo my morning coffee, but there are some things a man cannot do! I have always appreciated the jolt I get from a good cup of fully caffeinated coffee soon after I wake up.

When Az and I started working together, I followed a restricted diet. Not only was I trying to lose weight, but I was concerned about the type 2 diabetes I had recently been diagnosed with and knew a healthy diet would help control it. As it turned out, the diet and exercise put the diabetes into remission, so that now my blood sugar levels are normal and I feel great.

Slowly, we added foods to my weekly routine that are more in keeping with the way I eat now. The recipes in this book are not "diet" foods but rather wholesome dishes that taste good and are good for you. I pay close attention to the seasons and savor every fruit and vegetable when it is at its very best. As Az taught me, we all function best when we are healthy. Once you get your health under control—easier said than done for many people—the rest will flow.

Exercise Man

Az is the first to say that there is a lot of confusion in the health and fitness field. He believes that if even a little cardio exercise—walking, running, biking—were required for everyone in the workforce, we'd have a far more productive one. He cited a study where kids exercised for twenty minutes before class every day and their attention spans and ultimate test scores benefited.

I exercised for at least an hour a day when I was training with Az. This wasn't sissy stuff but hard, sweaty work. With his instruction and care, I never hurt myself but instead got stronger and more joyful every day.

His belief in the value of exercise was infectious. Now that Az is no longer part of my daily life, I sometimes goof off and skip a trip to the gym or a run around the neighborhood. But never for long. After even a day of missed exercise, my body craves it and I am back running or dancing on the treadmill, welcoming the attendant sweat, loose muscles, and exhilaration.

I am sure some people overdo exercise, but just as you can't eat too many vegetables, it's hard to exercise "too much." As my trainer explained, he burns about 600 calories an hour when he runs. And he is as fit as can be. Six hundred calories is not much; think how quickly you could eat 600 calories. A quarter-pound burger on a roll with cheese and ketchup is 800 calories, a slice of cheese pizza is 400 calories, and a fast-food hot fudge sundae is about 380. So, even if you are as fit and trim as Az, who does some sort of cardio exercise every day (running, cycling, or swimming) and resistance trains three times a week, you can't "just eat what you want."

Az remains a good and supportive friend. He has gone on to help others who need him more than I do, I am happy to say. Chicago trainer Joey Thurman has assumed the job of keeping Chef Art on track. I admit it's not always an easy task, but I am lucky to have Joey to jump-start my workouts and keep me moving and feeling great, along with my gym workout partner and friend, Ken Robling.

When you eat right, exercise regularly, and reclaim your good health, you won't turn to emotional eating—you won't need food to fill the void. Instead, you will be emotionally, mentally, and physically balanced, and life will become a lot easier and a lot more joyful. Can't beat it.

Breakfast: Start the Day Right!

Every morning I wake up knowing exactly what I will eat for breakfast, as I suspect many people do. The difference may be what we eat. I go for steel-cut oats (great fiber and nutrients), voluptuous lowfat or nonfat Greek yogurt (protein, calcium, pleasing texture), and some sort of seasonal fruit or berry (vitamins and natural sweetness). Believe me, this breakfast, which I have dubbed "Art Start," is about as good as it gets in terms of flavor, health, and satisfaction. (For more, see "Opting for Oatmeal" on page 17.) I often add an egg white to the mix for an extra boost of protein.

Breakfast is terribly important. Please don't skip it; you need to recharge your body after a good night's sleep to stay alert and be as productive as possible. This goes double for kids who are off to school. Equally important is *what* you eat. Too many of us have gotten in the habit of eating sugary cereals, donuts, and jam-laden toast for breakfast. We give our kids hot chocolate in the winter and pulp-free orange juice all year long. Many of us spoon sugar in our coffee and tea. None of these is a good idea. Too much sugar may give you a rush, but a few hours later, when you are sitting in a big meeting and your child has a math test, you'll both crash. Feel hungry and irritable, start counting the minutes until lunch, get a headache. Sound familiar?

By starting the day right with sugar-free foods that are high in protein, fiber, and carbohydrates that metabolize slowly, you will sail through the morning happily and productively, and four or five hours later you'll be ready for a good lunch. I hope you're convinced, because this surely is the most essential meal of the day.

Art Start Breakfast: Steel-Cut Oats with Greek Yogurt and Blueberries ❃ 15

Egg White Frittata with Roasted Mushrooms, Goat Cheese, and Basil ❃ 16

Breakfast Sandwich ❃ 18

Buckwheat Pancakes with Peaches and Greek Yogurt ❃ 20

Soft-Poached Egg and Root Vegetable Hash ❃ 22

Spinach-Feta Scramble with Lemon ❃ 24

Oatmeal and Quinoa Granola ❃ 26

Kale-Banana Smoothie ❃ 27

Blueberry-Peach Smoothie ❃ 28

Mango, Mint, and Pineapple Smoothie ❃ 29

Art Start Breakfast: Steel-Cut Oats with Greek Yogurt and Blueberries

~~~~~~

Here it is, the breakfast I most often start the day with. A version of it is on the menu at LYFE Kitchen, my restaurant in Northern California, as well as Art and Soul in Washington, D.C. You can substitute another berry or fruit for the blueberries, and if you are satisfied with the sweetness of the fruit, omit the honey or use less than called for here. However you fashion it, you'll love it!

Serves 4

1 cup steel-cut oats
Salt
¼ cup nonfat plain Greek yogurt
8 teaspoons honey
1 cup fresh blueberries
Grated zest of 1 lemon
4 mint leaves, chopped

METHOD Place the oatmeal in a preheated medium saucepan. Toast the oatmeal for 1 minute over medium-low heat, while stirring. Add 3½ cups water to the oatmeal. Bring to a simmer, reduce the heat to low, and cook the oatmeal for about 30 minutes, stirring every 5 minutes or so, or until the oatmeal is creamy and just cooked. Season to taste with salt.

ASSEMBLY Divide the cooked oatmeal among shallow bowls and spoon 1 tablespoon of Greek yogurt in the center of each serving. Drizzle 2 teaspoons of honey around the yogurt. Divide the berries among the bowls and top with the lemon zest. Sprinkle with the chopped mint.

Per serving: 146 calories • 1 g fat • 1 g sat fat • 0 mg chol • 43 mg sodium • 31 g carb • 16 g sugar • 3 g fiber • 4 g protein • 13 mg calcium

Egg White Frittata with Roasted Mushrooms, Goat Cheese, and Basil

~~~~~~

Looking for a protein punch to start the day? Try egg whites, which are nothing but protein. Here, they are shored up with goat cheese—another source of protein—and flavored with plenty of mushrooms and herbs. Our customers at LYFE Kitchen in Palo Alto, California, can't get enough of egg white frittatas.

Serves 4 to 6

For the frittata:
2 tablespoons extra-virgin olive oil
2 cups sliced cremini mushrooms
1 cup chopped Vidalia onion
1 garlic clove, chopped
12 large egg whites
2½ tablespoons chopped basil
Salt and freshly ground black pepper
3 tablespoons soft goat cheese

For the garnish:
4 basil leaves, chopped
Hot sauce (optional)

METHOD To prepare the frittata: Position a rack in the center of the oven and preheat to 350°F.

Place the olive oil in a preheated 10-inch nonstick sauté pan. Add the mushrooms and onions to the pan and cook over medium-high heat for about 4 minutes or until the onions are translucent and the mushrooms are cooked. Add the garlic to the pan and cook for 30 more seconds.

In a medium bowl, whisk the egg whites for 1 minute or until frothy. Add the basil and season with salt and pepper. Pour the egg white mixture over the mushroom mixture, and reduce the heat to medium-low. Drop small pieces of the goat cheese over the egg mixture and cook uncovered until the egg bottoms are just set, about 2 minutes. Transfer the skillet to the oven and bake for 10 to 12 minutes or until the frittata feels set when pressed in the center.

ASSEMBLY Invert the frittata onto a serving plate and slice into 4 to 6 pieces. Serve hot or cooled just to room temperature, topped with freshly ground black pepper, chopped basil, and hot sauce, if desired.

Per serving: 163 calories • 10 g fat • 3 g sat fat • 5 mg chol • 280 mg sodium • 6 g carb • 3 g sugar • 1 g fiber • 14 g protein • 43 mg calcium

Opting for Oatmeal

These days, I eat oatmeal most mornings. I remember liking it as a child, but it wasn't until I discovered steel-cut oats as a chef that I began to understand its culinary potential. A bowl of properly cooked oatmeal (see page 15 for my favorite recipe), festooned with some fruit and Greek yogurt or nuts, starts the day on a hopeful note. You know you are spooning good health into your body—and you also know you won't get hungry between now and lunch. How great is that?

There are dozens of reasons to eat oatmeal. It's high in soluble fiber and as such lowers levels of LDL ("bad") cholesterol even as it protects your HDL ("good") cholesterol. I can attest to this: I have normal cholesterol levels for my age.

Oatmeal is also credited with lowering the risk of certain cancers, including breast cancer. It may help reduce blood pressure and amps up your immune system. It's been shown to reduce the chance of developing type 2 diabetes because its high fiber content stabilizes blood glucose for hours. Again, I am living proof of this. Although I was diagnosed with type 2 diabetes in 2008, today my blood glucose levels are normal. I don't attribute this solely to oatmeal, but I bet it was a key factor. In fact, I believe a lot of my current good health comes from the oatmeal I eat just about every day.

I have sampled oatmeal in every city I have visited in the past three years. I have spooned it from bowls while sitting on hotel balconies in glamorous world capitals as well as in cramped diners along the road. When I eat it, I feel better all day long; my internal system is happier, and in turn so is my mood. It's not difficult to find a menu that offers oatmeal, and I am never sorry when I order it. Save the waffles, pancakes, and cinnamon buns for a party day brunch. Oatmeal rules! ※

Breakfast Sandwich

Served at LYFE Kitchen restaurant, this breakfast sandwich is perfect when you are on the run, and even better when enjoyed around the kitchen table with your family. Be sure to buy whole wheat muffins, a better source of complex carbs than the traditional English muffins.

Serves 4

4 1½-ounce turkey sausage patties
1 cup arugula, cleaned with large stems removed
2 teaspoons extra-virgin olive oil
6 large eggs
Salt and freshly ground black pepper
4 whole wheat English muffins, split and toasted
1 medium tomato, sliced

METHOD To prepare the turkey sausage and arugula: In a preheated small nonstick sauté pan, cook the turkey sausage patties over medium heat for 2 to 3 minutes on each side or until the patties are golden brown and thoroughly cooked. Remove the turkey sausage patties from the pan. Add the arugula to the same pan along with 1 tablespoon water. Quickly wilt the arugula and remove from the heat.

To prepare the eggs: Place the olive oil in a preheated nonstick medium sauté pan. Crack the eggs into a small mixing bowl and whisk together with a fork for 1 minute. Season with salt and freshly ground black pepper. Pour the egg mixture into the pan and let sit for 15 seconds. Using a small rubber spatula, gently move the eggs around the pan, scraping from the bottom every 7 seconds or so. Continue to cook the eggs for 2 minutes longer or until they are just cooked (they should glisten and be just set).

ASSEMBLY Place a cooked turkey sausage patty on each muffin bottom and top with the cooked eggs. Place the wilted arugula and sliced tomato over the eggs and top with the other half of the muffin. Serve immediately.

Per serving: 357 calories • 18 g fat • 3 g sat fat • 357 mg chol • 788 mg sodium • 30 g carb • 6 g sugar • 5 g fiber • 22 g protein • 216 mg calcium

Finding a Balance

One of the most valuable lessons I learned from Az is how crucial it is to find balance in your life. Being part of this planet is not an all-or-nothing endeavor. There are good times, great times, sad times, bad times, and boring times, and all of them need our attention. For example, our health can be fickle and bombard us with problems when we least expect it. These have to be addressed, but what's always true, Az says and I agree, is that our bodies want to support us in the best health possible.

Think of the most unhealthy person you know (and I don't mean someone who is actually ill). He or she is still living the life they always have, right? Sure, they may move a little slowly, may have trouble sleeping, may even smoke cigarettes, but overall their bodies are doing a Herculean job keeping them upright!

Take the same body and treat it right. Give it good, fresh food, plenty of exercise, and uninterrupted rest, and it will reward you with good health and a clear mind. I know it's not simplistic. People get sick regardless of what they do, but finding a balance in your life where you nourish your body and your mind will help you stay as healthy as you can.

I learned this the hard way when I was overweight and suffered from type 2 diabetes. I was on my way to a lifetime of failing health and doctor visits. No more! I have found balance in my life. I put staying healthy above all else because when you feel your best, you are your best.

I spent most of my adult life putting everyone else's needs before my own—foolish behavior that caused me a lot of stress and extra pounds. I was full of self-loathing and didn't think I was worth the attention others got. I was insecure about my overall self-worth and therefore tried to please everyone around me to affirm my value. Talk about convoluted reasoning!

Az arrived to help me control my weight and my health and ended up healing the whole man. I am dedicated to eating well, exercising regularly, and consequently feeling alert, in charge, contented, hopeful, and joyful. I never schedule a meeting or business call before my morning workout, yet my business runs more smoothly than ever! No personal or business issues before exercise is my mantra, and my personal life is happier for it. I have found emotional stability from this lifestyle, and once you find emotional stability, everything else falls into place and life is so much easier. Amen to that! ※

Buckwheat Pancakes
with Peaches and Greek Yogurt

Although I rarely indulge in pancakes anymore, when I get hold of buckwheat flour I can't resist making these. The peaches add a lovely flavor, and the thick, rich yogurt sweetened with a little maple syrup is the finishing touch.

Serves 4 to 6

For the pancakes:
1 cup buckwheat flour
1 cup whole wheat pastry flour
2 teaspoons baking powder
½ teaspoon baking soda
¼ teaspoon salt
2 large eggs, beaten
2½ cups buttermilk
1 teaspoon vanilla extract
2 peaches, peeled and cut into small dice
Cooking spray

For the garnish:
½ cup nonfat plain Greek yogurt
4 tablespoons maple syrup

METHOD Preheat the oven to 200°F.

In a large mixing bowl, combine the flours, baking powder, baking soda, and salt. In a separate medium mixing bowl, combine the eggs, buttermilk, and vanilla extract. Pour the egg mixture over the flour mixture and whisk until just combined. It is okay if there are still a few lumps. Fold in the peaches and set aside.

Preheat a griddle or large nonstick sauté pan over medium heat. Coat the surface with the cooking spray and pour ¼ cup batter into the pan for each pancake, leaving an inch between pancakes. Cook for 90 seconds on each side or until golden brown and cooked throughout. Transfer the pancakes to a parchment-lined baking sheet and hold in the oven. Repeat this process until you have used all the pancake batter.

ASSEMBLY Place 3 pancakes on each plate and top with 2 tablespoons of the Greek yogurt. Drizzle with 1 tablespoon of the maple syrup.

Per serving: 257 calories • 3 g fat • 1 g sat fat • 76 mg chol • 525 mg sodium • 46 g carb • 18 g sugar • 4 g fiber • 12 g protein • 201 mg calcium

Growing up we always cooked pancakes on a seasoned cast-iron griddle. There was a romance and a tradition to caring for the cast-iron pans that have been in my family for generations. Today in my home kitchen I often defer to cast iron, but when I want to cook with minimal oils I tend to use a high-quality nonstick pan. Nonstick pans really help make that perfect pancake, and they are a snap to clean!

Soft-Poached Egg and Root Vegetable Hash

Roasted root vegetables are one of the best things to come out of an oven. They are tender, boldly flavored, and seductively sweet. Pair them with poached eggs for a satisfying weekend breakfast. Here's a tip: double the amount of the veggies so you'll have leftovers to snack on.

Serves 4

For the root vegetable hash:
1 large sweet potato (2 cups), peeled and cut into medium dice
1 small rutabaga (1 cup), peeled and cut into medium dice
1 medium turnip (1 cup), peeled and cut into medium dice
1 small red onion, peeled and chopped
4 cloves garlic, minced
1½ tablespoons extra-virgin olive oil
Salt and freshly ground black pepper
2 tablespoons chopped flat-leaf parsley
2 tablespoons chopped basil
2 tablespoons fresh lemon juice

For the poached eggs:
2 teaspoons white wine vinegar
4 large eggs

METHOD To prepare the hash: Preheat the oven to 400°F.

In a large mixing bowl, combine the sweet potato, rutabaga, turnip, red onion, garlic, and olive oil. Season with salt and pepper. Spread the mixture on a large baking sheet or roasting pan. Roast while stirring occasionally for 50 to 60 minutes or until the vegetables are tender and caramelized. Stir in the parsley, basil, and lemon juice.

To prepare the eggs: Just prior to serving, bring a shallow saucepan of water to a simmer and add the vinegar. Crack each egg into a small cup and add to the simmering water one at a time. Poach the eggs for 1½ minutes, or until the whites are just set and the yolks are still soft. Gently remove the eggs from the water with a slotted spoon.

ASSEMBLY Spoon some root vegetable hash onto each plate and top with a poached egg. Garnish with freshly ground black pepper.

Per serving: 208 calories • 10 g fat • 2 g sat fat • 115 mg chol • 190 mg sodium • 23 g carb • 7 g sugar • 4 g fiber • 8 g protein • 84 mg calcium

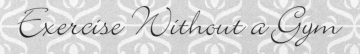

Exercise Without a Gym

You can't lose weight and keep it off without moving. And by moving, I mean exercising. For many of us who pack on the pounds, the idea of exercise is, well, threatening, unpleasant. "I don't want toooo," we whine. Can't we just skip dessert and pasta dinners and magically turn into a slim, gorgeous version of ourselves?

No. But you can have fun and feel great when you exercise.

Do what you like. If you prefer group classes for Zumba or aerobics, sign up. If you like to swim, join the local Y. If you are a walker, decide to walk farther. Jump rope! Join a softball league! Take up tennis! Just get out there and move. I promise: after a few weeks of sore muscles, you will be happy you pushed yourself, you'll start to look forward to your workouts, and your muscles will work smoothly without pain.

I started walking along Lake Michigan near my Chicago home. The walking soon turned into jogging, and that turned into running. You may want to stick with walking, which is fine. It's terrific exercise, but make sure you walk fast enough so your heart rate goes up and you are breathing hard enough that you can talk but not sing.

Speaking of singing, listening to music is a great way to inject your workout with energy. My friend Kenneth Robling programmed an iPod for me with hour-long music mixes. When the set was over, I knew my sixty-minute workout was over. Lady Gaga's "Born This Way" and "Bad Romance" from the Monster Ball tour helped me shake off more than fifty pounds as I propelled my way around the neighborhood. (Oprah's friend Gayle King added "Bad Romance" to her workout mix when I told her about it.) I even stopped in to see President Obama, who is a neighbor of mine. (Oprah introduced us!)

I am not wild about gyms. I find them a little lonely and cold, but there are times when they are a necessary part of a fitness program. When the weather is bad or I want to lift weights, I am off to the gym. One of my favorite gym workouts is to set the treadmill on a slow speed and then dance to the music playing in my ears. Other people at the gym may question my sanity, but who cares? I'm rocking out to get healthy. Yeah, baby! ❀

Spinach-Feta Scramble with Lemon

Who doesn't love scrambled eggs? Although there are three times as many egg whites as egg yolks in these, no one will notice, especially when the eggs are cooked with wilted spinach and kale topped with lemon-kissed feta cheese.

Serves 4

For the eggs:
4 large eggs
8 large egg whites
Salt and freshly ground black pepper

For the spinach:
2 teaspoons extra-virgin olive oil
½ cup chopped yellow onion
2 cups coarsely chopped baby spinach
1 cup coarsely chopped young kale

For the garnish:
½ teaspoon lemon juice
¼ teaspoon grated lemon zest
4 tablespoons crumbled feta cheese

METHOD In a medium mixing bowl, combine the eggs and egg whites. Whisk with a fork for 30 seconds until incorporated. Season with salt and pepper.

Heat the olive oil in a preheated nonstick large sauté pan over medium heat. Add the onion and cook for 2 minutes or until the onion is translucent. Add the spinach and kale and stir until the greens begin to wilt.

Add the egg mixture to the sauté pan with the wilted spinach and kale. Using a rubber spatula, move the eggs around the pan as you scramble to thoroughly combine them with the wilted spinach and kale. Cook over medium-high heat for 3 minutes or until the eggs are scrambled and just cooked.

ASSEMBLY Spoon the lemon juice over the scrambled eggs. Sprinkle with the lemon zest and feta cheese. Divide evenly over four plates.

Per serving: 168 calories • 9 g fat • 3 g sat fat • 223 mg chol • 379 mg sodium • 7 g carb • 2 g sugar • 1 g fiber • 16 g protein • 107 mg calcium

---

I love preparing breakfast and this is one of my weekend staples. Oftentimes I use kale or mustard greens in place of the spinach. You should have fun with this recipe. Try goat cheese in place of the feta, or crushed red pepper flakes for a little extra kick in the morning. If you have a small cast-iron pan you can make this into a frittata of sorts. There are no rules at breakfast!

Oatmeal and Quinoa Granola

~~~~~~

If you think granola is only for gym rats and mountain bikers, think again. Granola—so sweet, crunchy, and delicious—should be a staple of everyone's diet. A little goes a long way toward filling you up with good-for-you nuts and whole grains sweetened with stevia and a touch of honey. For more deliciousness, add dried fruits and unsweetened coconut, although they will add calories. Believe me, we can't keep enough of this at Art and Soul, my D.C. restaurant, or in my home kitchen. I bet you won't be able to either!

Serves 8

2 cups dried rolled oats
⅓ cup pecan halves
⅓ cup sliced almonds
¼ cup quinoa
¼ cup stevia
2 tablespoons honey
1 tablespoon molasses
½ teaspoon vanilla extract
¼ teaspoon ground cinnamon
Pinch of ground allspice
Pinch of ground coriander
Pinch of kosher salt

METHOD Preheat the oven to 325°F.

In a large mixing bowl, combine the oats, pecans, almonds, quinoa, stevia, honey, molasses, vanilla extract, cinnamon, allspice, coriander, and salt. Mix with a wooden spoon until the oats, nuts, and quinoa are well coated. Spread the oat mixture on a parchment-lined baking sheet.

Bake in the oven for 20 to 25 minutes, stirring the granola and rotating the baking sheet every 5 minutes.

Remove from the oven and allow to cool completely.

Store in an airtight container for up to 3 weeks.

Per serving: 169 calories • 7 g fat • 1 g sat fat • 0 mg chol • 16 mg sodium • 25 g carb • 7 g sugar • 3 g fiber • 5 g protein • 22 mg calcium

Kale-Banana Smoothie

You read right. Kale and bananas for a breakfast smoothie. Kale is packed with nutrients and fiber, and the banana, so sweet and creamy, gives the smoothie its body, while the apple juice makes it drinkable. Try it. You'll like it. It's a bestseller at LYFE Kitchen, my California restaurant, where Chef Jeremy Bringardner first created this smoothie.

Serves 1

1 cup chopped kale
1 frozen whole medium banana (about ⅔ cup pulp)
1 cup unfiltered apple juice
2-inch piece of cucumber
1 tablespoon lemon juice
¼ teaspoon chopped fresh ginger

METHOD Place all the ingredients in a blender with 2 ice cubes. Blend on high speed for about 60 seconds or until smooth.

ASSEMBLY Pour into a chilled glass and enjoy.

Per serving: 263 calories • 1 g fat • 0 g sat fat • 0 mg chol • 43 mg sodium • 64 g carb • 39 g sugar • 5 g fiber • 4 g protein • 124 mg calcium

Blueberry-Peach Smoothie

A traditional smoothie made with a generous amount of luxurious Greek yogurt is particularly good in the summer, when blueberries and peaches are at their best.

Serves 1

1 ripe peach, pitted and chopped
½ cup blueberries
½ cup nonfat high-protein plain Greek yogurt or kefir
2 teaspoons fresh lime juice

METHOD Place all the ingredients and 3 to 5 ice cubes in a blender and blend on high speed for about 60 seconds or until smooth.

ASSEMBLY Pour into a chilled glass and enjoy.

Per serving: 145 calories • 0 g fat • 0 g sat fat • 0 mg chol • 43 mg sodium • 26 g carb • 12 g sugar • 4 g fiber • 12 g protein • 81 mg calcium

$\mathcal{M}$ango, Mint, and Pineapple Smoothie

This smoothie transports you to the tropics with the mango and pineapple. I usually make it in my Chicago kitchen on a rainy day when I need some bright flavors.

Serves 1

½ cup chopped mango
½ cup chopped pineapple
½ cup nonfat high-protein plain Greek yogurt or kefir
4 mint leaves, torn into pieces

METHOD Place all the ingredients and 3 ice cubes in a blender and blend on high speed for about 60 seconds or until smooth.

ASSEMBLY Pour into a chilled glass and enjoy.

Per serving: 169 calories • 0 g fat • 0 g sat fat • 0 mg chol • 45 mg sodium • 33 g carb • 28 g sugar • 3 g fiber • 11 g protein • 97 mg calcium

4

First Courses and Snacks

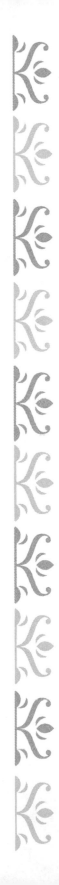

When I think of a first course, I think of a small plate of exquisitely prepared food. It might be a little rich, a tad indulgent, but because it's only a few bites, it's not only acceptable—it's treasured. Peppers stuffed with tangy goat cheese, shrimp paired with opulent avocado, and a lovely little tart with summer's best tomatoes and zucchini are all good examples. And so delicious, who can resist them? There's no reason to. No one prepares first courses on a regular basis; they are for special occasions, or perhaps you will indulge in one as a "main" course, and because a little goes a long way, you will feel totally satisfied.

Snacks are a different animal altogether. Sure, they are small bites of something tasty, but too many Americans think "salty" or "sweet" when they crave a snack. We eat far too many pretzels, chips, and candy bars. It's fine to snack between meals as long as you choose wisely. First, snacks should always be vegetarian, and they should never contain added sugar. Go for raw veggies, fruit, or a handful of raw nuts. All will satisfy your hunger, and you will feel better for choosing a juicy naval orange or the Oven-Dried Kale Chips on page 48 than you do after inhaling half a bag of tortilla chips.

Edamame Hummus with Cucumber Slices ✳ 33

Grilled Vegetable Antipasto with Balsamic Dressing ✳ 34

Shrimp and Avocado Ceviche ✳ 36

Spiced Raw Almonds ✳ 38

Tomatillo-Avocado Guacamole ✳ 39

Chicken Skewers with Cucumbers and Yogurt ✳ 40

Charred Eggplant Tapenade ✳ 42

Smoky Paprika-Baked Garbanzo Beans ✳ 43

Fire-Roasted Tomatillo Salsa and Baked Sprouted Corn Chips ✳ 44

Grilled Shisho Peppers Stuffed with Goat Cheese ✳ 46

Crab and Endive Salad ✳ 47

Oven-Dried Kale Chips ✳ 48

Art Smith's Healthy Comfort

Edamame Hummus with Cucumber Slices

The menu at LYFE Kitchen is loaded with vegetables, and this hummus is always a big hit. No surprise there, as I developed the menu with Tal Ronnen, the brilliant vegan chef. We make it with edamame, which are fresh soybeans, rather than the more expected chickpeas.

Serves 8 (1 quart)

1 pound frozen shelled edamame, thawed
½ cup tahini paste
¾ cup lemon juice
1½ tablespoons chopped garlic
2 teaspoons ground cumin
2 teaspoons ground coriander
½ cup extra-virgin olive oil
Salt
2 cucumbers, sliced ⅛ inch thick

METHOD In the bowl of a food processor fitted with a steel blade, mix the edamame, tahini, ½ cup water, lemon juice, garlic, cumin, and coriander and process until smooth. It may be necessary to stop the food processor and scrape down the sides of the bowl with a rubber spatula to ensure even mixing.

With the food processor running, slowly drizzle the oil into the hummus and process until fully incorporated. Season to taste with salt. Refrigerate the hummus until ready to serve.

ASSEMBLY Place the chilled edamame hummus in a serving bowl and set it alongside the sliced cucumbers.

Per serving: 289 calories • 25 g fat • 3 g sat fat • 0 mg chol • 10 mg sodium • 12 g carb • 3 g sugar • 4 g fiber • 9 g protein • 79 mg calcium

Grilled Vegetable Antipasto
with Balsamic Dressing

A platter of grilled veggies jazzed up with a little balsamic dressing is a wonderful way to start a summer meal. Plus, these are great snacks. The dressing can be used for salads, too.

Serves 4

For the balsamic dressing:
2 tablespoons balsamic vinegar
1 teaspoon Dijon mustard
⅓ cup extra-virgin olive oil
6 basil leaves, chopped
Salt and freshly ground black pepper

For the grilled vegetables:
2 zucchini
1 yellow squash
1 red bell pepper
12 asparagus stalks
8 green onions, cleaned
4 stalks rapini (also called broccoli rabe)

For the garnish:
4 basil leaves, chopped

METHOD To prepare the dressing: In a mason jar with a lid, combine the balsamic vinegar, Dijon mustard, olive oil, and chopped basil. Secure the lid and shake for 1 minute or until the oil and vinegar are combined. Season to taste with salt and pepper.

To prepare the antipasto: Preheat a grill to moderate heat.

Slice the zucchini and yellow squash into ⅛-inch-thick lengthwise slices. Cut the bell pepper into quarters and remove the seeds. Trim the ends of the asparagus. In a large mixing bowl, combine the zucchini, yellow squash, bell pepper, asparagus, green onions, and rapini. Pour half the balsamic dressing over the vegetables and toss until combined.

Arrange the vegetables on the grill over medium heat. Cook the vegetables for 2 minutes on each side or until they have a nice char and are just cooked. Remove from the grill and cool to room temperature.

ASSEMBLY Arrange the vegetables on a large platter. Just prior to serving, drizzle lightly with the remaining balsamic dressing and sprinkle with the remaining chopped basil.

Per serving: 231 calories • 19 g fat • 3 g sat fat • 0 mg chol • 57 mg sodium • 14 g carb • 7 g sugar • 4 g fiber • 5 g protein • 75 mg calcium

Shrimp and Avocado Ceviche

In case you are not sure about this, the acid from the lime juice "cooks" the shrimp, even as it flavors the avocados, onion, and cucumber. I love the jolt of heat from the jalapeno, but if you prefer your food mild, leave it out.

Serves 8

16 raw jumbo shrimp, peeled, deveined, and cut into bite-size pieces
2 avocados, cut into medium chunks
¾ cup chopped red onion
1 cucumber, peeled, seeded, and cut into medium dice
1 jalapeno pepper, seeded and minced (optional)
1½ tablespoons extra-virgin olive oil
Juice of 3 limes
Salt
¼ cup chopped cilantro leaves (thick stalks discarded)
16 small leaves butter lettuce

METHOD In a medium mixing bowl, combine the shrimp, avocado, red onion, cucumber, jalapeno, olive oil, and lime juice. Stir gently to ensure even mixing. Cover with plastic wrap and refrigerate for 1 hour. Remove from the refrigerator, season to taste with salt, and fold in the chopped cilantro.

ASSEMBLY Spoon some of the chilled ceviche onto each butter lettuce leaf and arrange on a serving platter.

Per serving: 105 calories • 8 g fat • 1 g sat fat • 21 mg chol • 29 mg sodium • 7 g carb • 2 g sugar • 3 g fiber • 4 g protein • 22 mg calcium

Travel Is for Exercise

You may have a convenient and easy-to-follow exercise routine when you are home, but when you travel it falls apart. Does this matter? If you travel infrequently, probably not so much, but if you are like me, climbing on and off planes week in and week out, working exercise into your day is key.

Running or walking is easy to "take on the road." All you need are your running shoes, although running clothes and a well-programmed iPod help, too. When I stay in unfamiliar hotels, I ask the concierge or someone at the desk to point me in the right direction for a run. It's a joy to wake up in a new city and take a quick tour of its parks, waterfront, or urban streets. When I am in familiar cities, I already know where to go, and it's heartening to run the same routes and get reacquainted with the neighborhood.

You might prefer using the hotel gym. If you walk, keep up a good pace and resist the temptation to stroll. If you use the gym, do both cardio and weight training, although if time is short, concentrate on the cardio.

If you have some downtime, look into renting a bike. Find out where the best nearby hiking trails are. See if you can rent a kayak if you are near a lake or river. Many local health clubs sell short-term memberships or have arrangements with local hotels. This way you can swim laps, join a class, or just use the facilities. These activities are fun as well as good for you.

Why exercise when you travel? Simple. You will feel better. Negotiating airports and cities can be stressful—you can overeat or eat the "wrong food." If it's business travel, you might be anxious about a presentation or meeting. Our digestive tracts don't always work well when we're away from home, muscles may ache from hoisting luggage, and our sleep patterns are interrupted. Believe it or not, exercise helps all of these. Let's hear it for exercise (once again!). ❄

Spiced Raw Almonds

All nuts are good for you, and almonds are the best. "Good" fats, omega-3 fatty acids, protein, and fiber are all there, plus an ounce of the tasty treats supplies half the vitamin E a healthy adult needs every day. Why care about vitamin E? It's an important antioxidant and we all need it, that's why! Raw nuts are easier to metabolize, I find, and when I spice 'em up, they are even more tempting.

Serves 12 (2 cups)

¼ teaspoon chili powder
¼ teaspoon curry powder
¼ teaspoon garlic powder
½ teaspoon stevia
3 tablespoons low-sodium soy sauce
2 cups whole raw almonds

METHOD In a medium mixing bowl, combine the chili powder, curry powder, garlic powder, stevia, soy sauce, and almonds. Toss with a spoon until fully combined. Store in an airtight container until ready to use.

Another way to prepare the nuts is to spread the seasoned almonds on a baking sheet and bake in the oven at 325°F for about 20 minutes or until the almonds are golden brown and fragrant.

Per serving: 140 calories • 12 g fat • 1 g sat fat • 0 mg chol • 134 mg sodium • 6 g carb • 1 g sugar • 3 g fiber • 5 g protein • 64 mg calcium

Tomatillo-Avocado Guacamole

Avocados are really good for you, although no one denies that their heart-healthy monounsaturated fat can add calories to your diet. So how to include these nutritious powerhouses? Eat them in small amounts, and what better way than as guacamole? This is one of my favorite recipes for the dip/condiment. Tomatillos, which grow in the same climate as avocados, have enough acid to keep the guac from oxidizing and turning brown. Make this up to a day ahead of time and store in the fridge, tightly covered.

Serves 4

2 tomatillos, husk removed, quartered
2 avocados, peeled, pit removed, and chopped
Juice of 2 limes
½ cup minced white onion
1 jalapeno, seeded and minced
¼ cup chopped cilantro, thick stalks discarded
Salt

METHOD Place the tomatillos, chopped avocado, and lime juice in a food processor and puree until smooth. Fold in the onion, jalapeno, and cilantro. Season with salt.

ASSEMBLY Transfer the guacamole to a serving bowl and refrigerate until ready to serve.

Per serving: 134 calories • 11 g fat • 1 g sat fat • 0 mg chol • 7 mg sodium • 11 g carb • 2 g sugar • 5 g fiber • 2 g protein • 18 mg calcium

Chicken Skewers with Cucumbers and Yogurt

Little skewers of grilled chicken served with a classic Greek cucumber and yogurt salad make appealing appetizers or even a light meal. The salad, or side dish, known as tzatziki and made with cukes, lemon juice, and dill, is a cool accompaniment to the chicken or any other grilled meat. The tzatziki can be made a day ahead of time, covered, and refrigerated.

Serves 4

For the cucumbers and yogurt:
2 cucumbers, peeled and seeded
2 cups nonfat Greek yogurt
2 garlic cloves, peeled and chopped
3 tablespoons lemon juice
2 tablespoons dill, chopped
Salt

For the chicken:
2 skinless and boneless chicken breasts
1 tablespoon extra-virgin olive oil
Salt
12 bamboo skewers, soaked in water

METHOD To prepare the cucumbers: Grate the cucumbers using a handheld grater on the side with the large holes. Place the grated cucumber in a mixing bowl and, using your hands, squeeze out the excess cucumber juice. Discard (or drink) the cucumber juice and return the grated cucumber to the bowl. Add the yogurt, garlic, lemon juice, and dill. Stir until incorporated and season with salt. Cover and refrigerate until ready to use.

To prepare the chicken skewers: Preheat a grill to moderate heat.

Cut each of the chicken breasts into 6 strips. Place the chicken strips in a mixing bowl. Toss with the olive oil and season lightly with salt. Thread a chicken strip on each bamboo skewer. Grill the chicken skewers for 2 to 3 minutes on each side or until just cooked. Remove from the grill. Serve either warm or at room temperature.

ASSEMBLY Place the cucumber and yogurt mixture in a serving bowl. Arrange the grilled chicken skewers on a serving platter and serve alongside the cucumber and yogurt.

Per serving: 178 calories • 5 g fat • 1 g sat fat • 37 mg chol • 77 mg sodium • 8 g carb • 6 g sugar • 1 g fiber • 24 g protein • 100 mg calcium

What Are the Best Snacks?

The best snacks are those you like and that satisfy a craving, but not a craving so indulgent that you decide to snack on ice cream with hot fudge sauce and whipped cream! If you feel like something sweet, snack on fruit. If you want something salty, grab a handful of nuts.

Everyone's metabolism is slightly different. But when it comes to snacking, less is always better, and yet often is key. Confused? What I mean is, snack when you're hungry but never eat too much. Don't let hunger so consume you that you toss caution to the wind when you come across a well-stocked refrigerator. Snack often so that you never feel ravenous. On the other hand, you should never feel stuffed. Moderation, folks. Moderation!

Az, my health coach, taught me to make shakes using nonfat yogurt and sweet, ripe, juicy fruit. For a savory snack, I like to dip raw veggies, like carrots, celery, and broccoli, into a yogurt-based dip. Other favorites? Protein shakes, raw almonds, string cheese. ❈

Charred Eggplant Tapenade

~~~~~~

Classic Provençal tapenade is made with olives, garlic, and lots of olive oil. I love it but have discovered how to make a similar spread with far fewer calories. I use grilled eggplant, mixed with yogurt and cumin, for a totally delectable alternative. Serve it as a spread on toasted pita bread or crackers, or as an accompaniment to lamb, chicken, or beef. The tapenade can be made a day in advance.

Serves 4

1 large (14-ounce) eggplant
⅓ cup nonfat Greek yogurt
1 teaspoon ground cumin
1 tablespoon extra-virgin olive oil
1 tablespoon lemon juice
Salt

METHOD Preheat a grill to moderate heat.

Place the whole eggplant on the grill and cook for 10 minutes on each side or until the entire eggplant is charred and tender. Remove the eggplant from the grill and let cool to room temperature.

Cut the eggplant open and spoon the flesh into a sieve set over a bowl. Drain for 1 hour. Transfer the eggplant to a bowl and mash with a fork. Add the yogurt, cumin, olive oil, and lemon juice and stir until fully incorporated. Season with salt. Refrigerate until ready to serve.

Per serving: 76 calories • 4 g fat • 1 g sat fat • 0 mg chol • 11 mg sodium • 9 g carb • 4 g sugar • 5 g fiber • 3 g protein • 29 mg calcium

Smoky Paprika-Baked Garbanzo Beans

~~~~~~

These jazzy little beans are hard to stop popping in your mouth—and they are so easy to make it's almost ludicrous to call this a recipe. I often have some around to snack on. Big taste, little damage!

Serves 4

30 ounces canned garbanzo beans, drained
1 tablespoon smoked paprika
1 teaspoon onion powder

METHOD Preheat the oven to 350°F.

In a medium mixing bowl, toss the drained garbanzo beans with the smoked paprika and onion powder. Spread the beans on a parchment-lined baking sheet. Bake for 1 hour, stirring occasionally, until the beans are browned and crisp. Remove from the oven and cool the beans to room temperature. Store in an airtight container until ready to enjoy.

Per serving: 176 calories • 3 g fat • 0 g sat fat • 0 mg chol • 474 mg sodium • 30 g carb • 3 g sugar • 7 g fiber • 9 g protein • 39 mg calcium

Fire-Roasted Tomatillo Salsa and Baked Sprouted Corn Chips

~~~~~~~~~~~~~~~~~~~~~~~~~~~~~~~~

It really is easy to make your own oven-baked corn chips—ten minutes and they are done. The chips beg for a salsa for dipping, so I devised this simple one using mildly tangy tomatillos mixed with lime juice, onions, and cilantro. Tomatillos are sometimes called Mexican tomatoes and come with a papery brown husk that needs to be removed before they can be grilled.

Serves 8

For the salsa:
10 medium tomatillos
Juice of 2 limes
1 small white onion, chopped
1 serrano chile pepper, seeded and finely minced
¼ cup cilantro leaves, chopped
Salt

For the corn chips:
Twelve 8-inch yellow or blue sprouted corn tortillas
1 lime

METHOD To prepare the salsa: Preheat an outdoor grill to a moderate heat.

Remove the husks from the tomatillos and grill them for 5 minutes on each side or until they have a nice char on the outside skin. Remove from the grill and let cool to room temperature.

Put the tomatillos and lime juice in the blender or food processor and puree until smooth. Transfer to a serving bowl and fold in the onion, serrano chile pepper, and cilantro. Season to taste with salt.

To prepare the corn chips: Preheat the oven to 350°F.

Cut each of the corn tortillas into 6 triangles. Place on a parchment-lined baking sheet, making sure that they only overlap slightly. Bake in the oven for 10 minutes or until the corn tortillas begin to crisp up. Remove from the oven.

ASSEMBLY Place the baked corn tortillas in a serving bowl and squeeze the lime over the chips just prior to serving. Serve alongside the Fire-Roasted Tomatillo Salsa.

Per serving: 104 calories • 2 g fat • 0 g sat fat • 0 mg chol • 1 mg sodium • 21 g carb • 2 g sugar • 3 g fiber • 3 g protein • 52 mg calcium

Don't Drink Your Calories

Oddly enough, many of us think more about the calories in the food we eat than in what we drink. I had to remind myself often when I started losing weight that while it was important to keep hydrated, the best choice was and always will be water. Plain tap water, sparkling water, and water flavored with a little lemon or lime are all great choices when you are thirsty. This doesn't mean you can never drink anything else, but if you put water at the top of the list, you can't go wrong.

I like to have a cocktail now and then, but don't be fooled into thinking that the gin and tonic sliding so effortlessly down your throat is a freebie. It has about 160 calories. A cup of orange juice has 112 calories, and a can of soda 165. See what I mean about drinking calories?

Many trainers and weight-loss coaches suggest you never drink alcohol. It lowers your resistance, so you are apt to throw caution to the wind and order a second drink. I don't subscribe to this all-or-nothing approach. To me, it's like saying no more chocolate for the rest of your life. I postpone having wine or vodka until my weekly party (or free) day. And then I drink only one glass and never think about a second. ✳

Grilled Shisho Peppers
Stuffed with Goat Cheese

~~~~~~

Like mild-flavored poppers, these tiny, mild peppers are stuffed with cheese and then grilled. Use any small, mild peppers if you can't find shishos. Take care, though, as many small peppers are fiery.

Serves 4

24 shisho peppers or other small, green mild peppers
1½ tablespoons extra-virgin olive oil
4 ounces soft goat cheese
Salt

METHOD Preheat an outdoor grill to moderate heat.

In a medium mixing bowl, toss the peppers with the olive oil. Cut a slit in each pepper near the stem end to create an opening; do not go through both sides. Using your fingers, press a pinch of goat cheese into the opening of the pepper. Continue this process until you have stuffed all 24 peppers with the goat cheese.

Place the stuffed peppers on the grill over a medium flame. Grill the peppers for 1 minute on each side or until the peppers have a nice char on them. Remove from the grill and season with salt.

ASSEMBLY Place the grilled shisho peppers in a serving bowl and enjoy immediately.

Per serving: 229 calories • 12 g fat • 5 g sat fat • 13 mg chol • 123 mg sodium • 26 g carb • 14 g sugar • 4 g fiber • 11 g protein • 88 mg calcium

Crab and Endive Salad

Superluxurious crabmeat is made even more so with the addition of a little sour cream to augment the yogurt. Once the salad is made, eat it as finger food nestled in long, curved endive leaves. This is a treat anytime and a perfect party dish, too. If you are planning to serve it to guests, don't make it more than three hours ahead of time.

Serves 8

12 ounces lump crabmeat, shell pieces removed
1 stalk celery, finely chopped
½ cup finely chopped red bell pepper
⅓ cup nonfat Greek yogurt
2 tablespoons nonfat sour cream
2 tablespoons lemon juice
1 tablespoon fresh lime juice
1 tablespoon chopped fresh tarragon
Salt
1 medium avocado, peeled, pit removed, and diced
16 endive leaves

METHOD In a medium mixing bowl, combine the crabmeat, celery, red pepper, yogurt, sour cream, lemon juice, lime juice, and tarragon. Mix until thoroughly combined. Season with salt and gently fold in the avocado. Refrigerate until ready to serve.

ASSEMBLY Place 2 tablespoons of the crab mixture into each endive leaf and arrange on a serving platter.

Per serving: 94 calories • 3 g fat • 0 g sat fat • 30 mg chol • 185 mg sodium • 6 g carb • 2 g sugar • 3 g fiber • 11 g protein • 82 mg calcium

Oven-Dried Kale Chips

Addiction alert! Once you start eating these crunchy, crispy chips you won't be able to stop! No worries: they are low in calories and high in nutritive value. I add a little nutritional yeast (also known as vegetarian support supplement—an unappealing name!—or nooch, for some reason) for the B-complex vitamins, folic acid, and protein and for the pungent punch it adds to the kale's flavor.

Serves 4

1 bunch kale (about 8 ounces)
1 tablespoon extra-virgin olive oil
1 teaspoon nutritional yeast
¼ teaspoon cayenne
Salt

METHOD Preheat the oven to 350°F.

Strip the kale leaves off the thick stalks and discard the stalks. Wash the kale leaves and dry in a salad spinner. In a large mixing bowl, toss the leaves with the olive oil, nutritional yeast, and cayenne. Season with salt.

Lay the kale leaf pieces on a parchment-lined baking sheet, being careful not to overlap or crowd the pieces. If necessary use an additional baking sheet. Bake for 15 to 20 minutes or until the kale is crispy but not beginning to burn. Remove from the oven and allow to cool completely. Store in an airtight container until ready to use. If your chips get a bit soft, you can crisp them up again in the oven.

Per serving: 61 calories • 4 g fat • 1 g sat fat • 0 mg chol • 25 mg sodium • 6 g carb • 0 g sugar • 1 g fiber • 2 g protein • 77 mg calcium

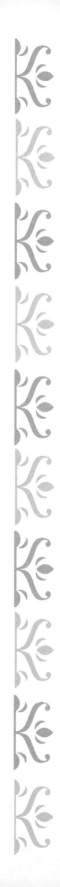

5

Soups

ew people get fat from soup! It's hard to shovel in big spoonfuls of hot liquid; rather, its consistency demands that you eat it carefully, a little slowly, so that despite yourself you end up savoring it fully. It's a complete meal, easily digestible and bursting with any flavor you especially like. If you must eat late in the evening, make it a bowl of vegetable soup. When lunch has been unavoidably delayed and it's inching close to the dinner hour, stave off your hunger with a cup of soup. It works every time.

Most of the time, I prefer simple vegetable soups packed with the best seasonal veggies in the market. On cold days, I might add a few ounces of cooked chicken to the vegetables. In the summer, I like to make gazpacho. Just eating it makes me feel healthy! Chunkier soups, such as the Curried Cauliflower Soup on page 58 and Three-Bean Turkey Chili on page 55 (which arguably is more of a stew than a soup, but why quibble—it tastes amazing!), are whole meals that need nothing more than a plain green salad to round them out. Making your own soup is ridiculously easy once you realize that "anything goes" and you won't make a mistake by adding green beans instead of snow peas,

Swiss chard in place of spinach. When you know you have a pot of homemade soup waiting for you in the refrigerator, you happily anticipate your next meal—and are far less apt to grab an unhealthy snack to munch in the car on the way home.

Yellow Tomato Gazpacho ❈ 51

Melon Soup with Grilled Shrimp ❈ 52

White Bean Soup with Kale and Turkey Andouille Sausage ❈ 54

Three-Bean Turkey Chili ❈ 55

Sweet Corn Soup with Cilantro ❈ 57

Curried Cauliflower Soup ❈ 58

Miso Corn Chowder ❈ 60

Roasted Sweet Potato and Ginger Soup ❈ 61

Frogmore Stew ❈ 62

Lentil and Escarole Soup with Manchego Cheese ❈ 63

Jambalaya ❈ 65

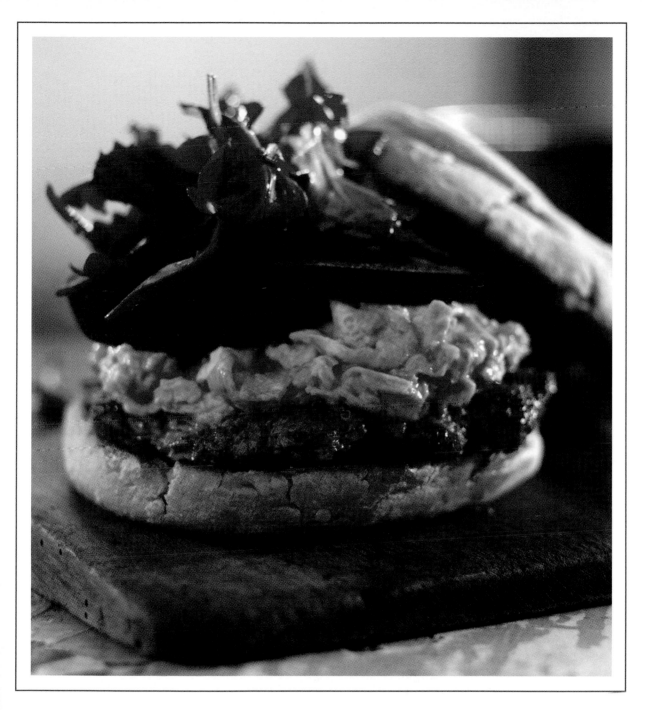

❋ BREAKFAST SANDWICH (page 18) ❋

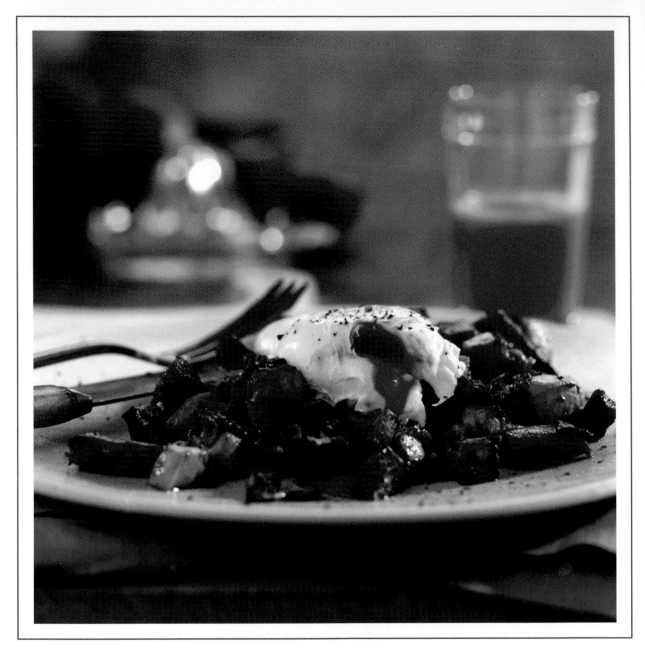

❋ SOFT-POACHED EGG AND ROOT VEGETABLE HASH (page 22) ❋

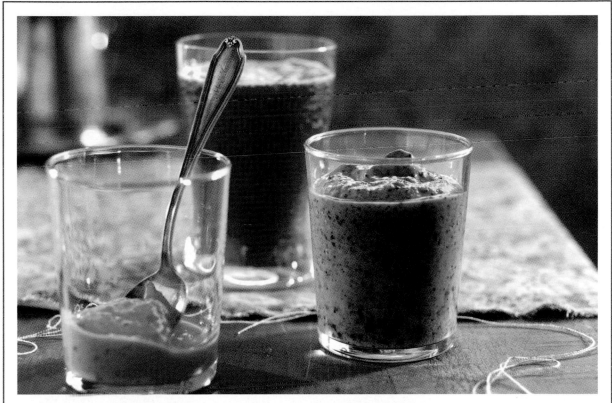

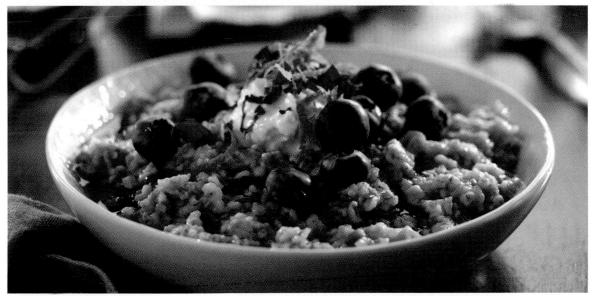

※ *Top:* MANGO, MINT, AND PINEAPPLE SMOOTHIE (page 29); KALE-BANANA SMOOTHIE
(page 27); BLUEBERRY-PEACH SMOOTHIE (page 28) ※
※ *Bottom:* ART START BREAKFAST: STEEL-CUT OATS WITH
GREEK YOGURT AND BLUEBERRIES (page 15) ※

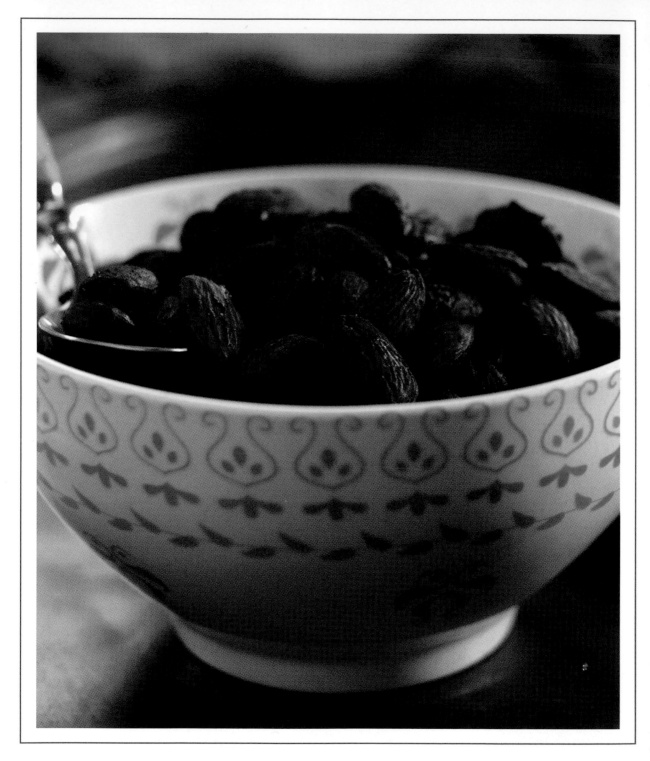

❈ SPICED RAW ALMONDS (page 38) ❈

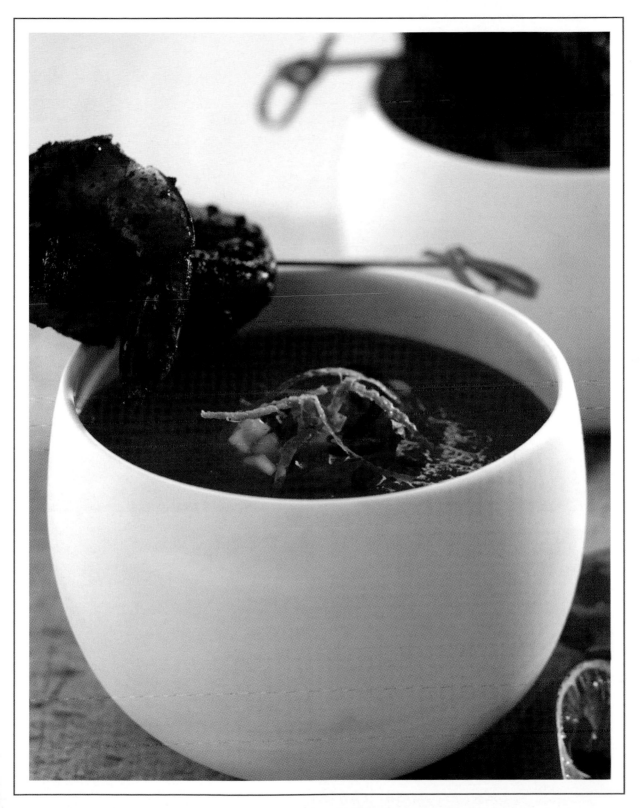

❋ MELON SOUP WITH GRILLED SHRIMP (page 52) ❋

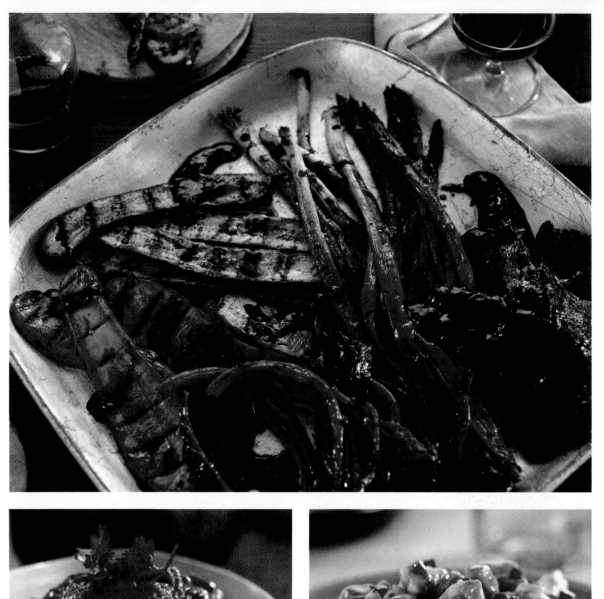

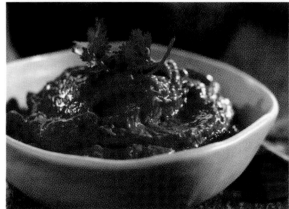

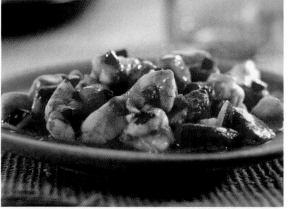

❊ *Top:* GRILLED VEGETABLE ANTIPASTO WITH BALSAMIC DRESSING (page 34) ❊
❊ *Lower left:* TOMATILLO-AVOCADO GUACAMOLE (page 39) ❊
❊ *Lower right:* SHRIMP AND AVOCADO CEVICHE (page 36) ❊

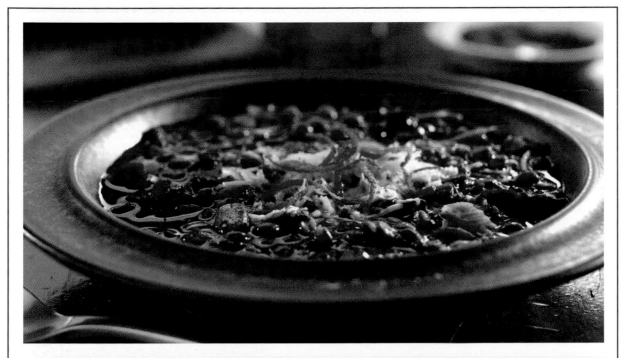

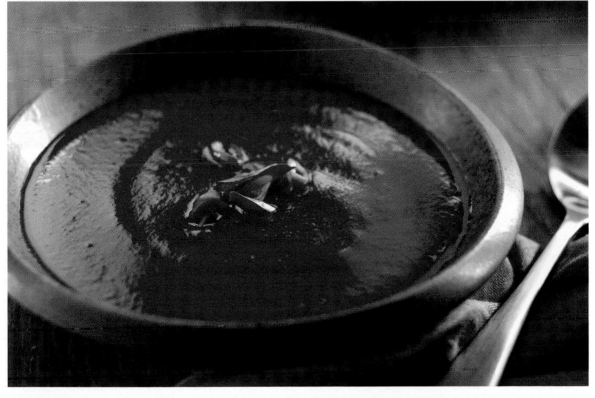

❋ *Top:* LENTIL AND ESCAROLE SOUP WITH MANCHEGO CHEESE (page 63) ❋
❋ *Bottom:* ROASTED SWEET POTATO AND GINGER SOUP (page 61) ❋

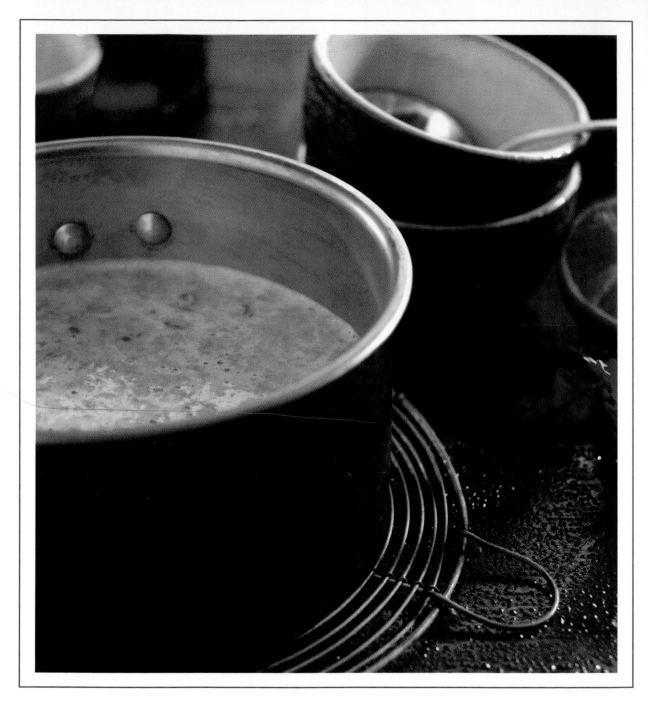

❋ SWEET CORN SOUP WITH CILANTRO (page 57) ❋

Yellow Tomato Gazpacho

There's something about the deep, golden color of yellow tomatoes that makes this gazpacho look as refreshing as it tastes. If you can't find them, use whatever tomatoes you can get hold of, as long as they are fresh and fragrant, tasting of summer's sunshine. On a party day, strain the soup and add a little vodka for a killer Bloody Mary.

Serves 4

For the gazpacho:
2½ pounds ripe yellow tomatoes, chopped
1 cucumber, peeled, seeded, and chopped
1 jalapeno, seeded and chopped
1 yellow bell pepper, seeded and chopped
2 cloves garlic, coarsely chopped
½ cup minced red onion
3 tablespoons extra-virgin olive oil
2 tablespoons red wine vinegar
Salt and freshly ground black pepper

For the garnish:
8 basil leaves, chopped
4 teaspoons olive oil (optional)

METHOD In the bowl of a food processer fitted with a metal blade, puree the tomatoes, cucumber, jalapeno, bell pepper, garlic, and onion. Add the olive oil, vinegar, and 6 ice cubes and puree until almost smooth. Season with salt and pepper.

Remove from the food processor and serve immediately or refrigerate for 30 minutes or until chilled. (For a smoother soup, strain through a sieve.)

ASSEMBLY Divide the gazpacho among 4 chilled serving bowls and sprinkle with the chopped basil and extra olive oil if desired.

Per serving (without optional olive oil): 164 calories • 11 g fat • 2 g sat fat • 0 mg chol • 69 mg sodium • 15 g carb • 3 g sugar • 3 g fiber • 4 g protein • 53 mg calcium

$\mathcal{M}$elon Soup with Grilled Shrimp

The Japanese know a thing or two when it comes to seasoning seafood, and togarashi is a spice blend that makes the shrimp used here the perfect accompaniment for this supercooling melon soup. Togarashi is salt-free and often found on the dinner table in Japan, where it is sprinkled liberally over any number of foods. I like it with shrimp, but it's also great with fish, poultry, and beef. It's showing up more often in the Asian section of supermarkets and can be found in Asian groceries and some specialty stores.

Serves 4

For the soup:
1 large cantaloupe, peeled, seeded, and cut into medium cubes
Juice of 1 lemon
2 tablespoons extra-virgin olive oil
Salt and freshly ground black pepper

For the shrimp:
8 large shrimp, peeled and deveined
1 tablespoon extra-virgin olive oil
½ teaspoon togarashi spice
Salt
4 bamboo skewers, soaked in water

For the garnish:
¼ cup minced cucumber
1 Thai red chili, thinly sliced
4 teaspoons chopped fresh mint
Grated zest of 1 lemon

METHOD **To prepare the soup:** Place the cantaloupe, lemon juice, and olive oil in a food processor fitted with a metal blade, and puree until smooth. Season with salt and pepper and refrigerate for 1 hour.

To prepare the shrimp: Preheat a grill to moderate heat.

In a medium mixing bowl, toss together the shrimp, olive oil, and togarashi spice and season with salt. Place 2 shrimp on each skewer.

Cook the prepared shrimp on the grill for 2 minutes on each side or until just cooked. Remove from the grill and cool to room temperature.

ASSEMBLY Divide the soup equally among 4 chilled serving bowls. Sprinkle the cucumber, Thai red chili, mint, and lemon zest over the soup. Lay a bamboo skewer over each bowl and serve.

Per serving: 180 calories • 11 g fat • 2 g sat fat • 21 mg chol • 59 mg sodium • 19 g carb • 16 g sugar • 2 g fiber • 4 g protein • 31 mg calcium

White Bean Soup with Kale and Turkey Andouille Sausage

~~~~~~

Without question, this is a soup that hits the spot on a cold, blustery day—and where I come from, it gets cold and blustery! Full of bold, full flavors, the white beans can handle eight cloves of garlic and Andouille sausage, so the final result is perfectly balanced.

Serves 6

For the soup:
2 tablespoons extra-virgin olive oil
1 large yellow onion, chopped
8 garlic cloves, smashed
5 cups low-sodium chicken stock
6 ounces kale, cleaned
2 cans (15 ounces each) cannellini beans, drained and rinsed
½ pound smoked turkey andouille sausage, sliced ¼ inch thick
Salt and freshly ground black pepper

For the garnish:
4 tablespoons grated pecorino Romano cheese

METHOD Heat the oil in a large saucepan over medium heat. Add the onion to the pan and cook for 4 to 5 minutes over medium heat or until translucent. Add the garlic and stock to the saucepan and bring to a simmer.

Trim the thick stems from the kale and tear or chop the leaves into 1-inch pieces. Add the kale and beans to the saucepan. Simmer the soup for 15 minutes or until the kale is fully wilted and the beans are tender. Add the turkey andouille sausage to the soup and cook for 15 minutes or until the sausage is hot and the flavors come together. Season with salt and pepper.

ASSEMBLY Divide the soup among 6 serving bowls and sprinkle 2 teaspoons of pecorino Romano cheese over each bowl.

Per serving: 303 calories • 11 g fat • 3.5 g sat fat • 29 mg chol • 867 mg sodium • 32 g carb • 4 g sugar • 7.5 g fiber • 22 g protein • 185 mg calcium

Three-Bean Turkey Chili

I had to include this wonderful recipe because it's so darn good. Who doesn't love chili? I know it's not exactly a soup, but it's cooked in a big pot and holds its own as a full meal, so I decided it could be slipped in here. And once you make it, you'll be glad I did! If it's been a while since you made chili, replace the chili powder that has been languishing in your cupboard. Fresh chili powder has more "umph," and the stew will be far tastier.

Serves 8

For the chili:
2 tablespoons extra-virgin olive oil
2 pounds ground turkey
2 tablespoons chili powder
1 tablespoon ground smoked paprika
1 tablespoon ground cumin
1 large onion, chopped
4 garlic cloves, chopped
2 18-ounce jars or cans stewed, chopped tomatoes
1 15-ounce can black beans, drained
1 15-ounce can kidney beans, drained
1 15-ounce can cannellini beans, drained
3 tablespoons balsamic vinegar
1 tablespoon hot sauce
Salt

For the garnish:
8 tablespoons chopped cilantro or chives

METHOD Heat the olive oil in a large Dutch oven or soup pot over medium-high heat. Add the ground turkey, chili powder, paprika, and cumin. Cook for 6 to 8 minutes, stirring occasionally, or until the turkey is cooked.

Add the onion, garlic, tomatoes, black beans, kidney beans, cannellini beans, balsamic vinegar, and hot sauce to the pot and bring to a simmer. Cook over medium-low heat for 45 minutes or until all the flavors have married. Season with salt.

ASSEMBLY Divide the chili among 8 serving bowls and sprinkle with the chopped cilantro or chives.

Per serving: 389 calories • 12 g fat • 3 g sat fat • 65 mg chol • 736 mg sodium • 40 g carb • 8 g sugar • 12 g fiber • 34 g protein • 106 mg calcium

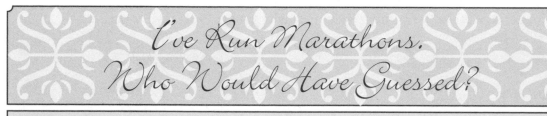

I've Run Marathons, Who Would Have Guessed?

Before I decided to change the way I lived, ate, and exercised, I would have scoffed at the idea of running a marathon. Me? Run for more than twenty-six miles without stopping? Forget it! I couldn't run a mile.

As I've said, I was especially fortunate to find Az Ferguson to coach me through it all. Az was there when I was convinced I could not go on *for one more day!* He was there to celebrate, too, when I passed another milestone. You may not have an Az in your life, but you probably have a husband or wife, best friend, sister, or brother who could be there for you—or you could be there for each other. Even better.

As I told you, I started out walking. After a while, walking became jogging. Jogging morphed into running, and before I knew it, I was running through the park along Lake Michigan, covering three miles, five miles, six miles. Hey, I discovered, I love to run!

It wasn't long until I was training for the Chicago Marathon. My family doctor and dear friend, Dr. Jeffrey Raizer, gave me the green light to train in earnest, and as I did I just got healthier. On race day, I was ner-vous, but running through the streets of my beloved adopted city was a joy. Az ran with me and monitored my heart rate as we went along. As exciting as it was, it was also difficult. Believe me, by mile 18, it's hard to find that happy place! Thanks to Az urging me on, the crowd cheering as I ran by, and television crews who took great delight in documenting Chef Art huffing and puffing mile after mile, I made it. And I finished in the top ten thousand, which isn't too shabby considering there were more than thirty thousand runners.

I also ran the Marine Corps Marathon, and I am proud to say that I beat Oprah's time. I ran the Magellan Half Marathon to benefit the Northwestern Brain Tumor Institute, a race I was particularly proud to run because Dr. Raizer also runs in it. And I have run in two 10Ks and happily placed in my age group. As you can tell, I am totally into this running gig.

You may not be as captivated by running or any other sport, but when you decide to lose weight and feel better, my advice is to surround yourself with people who love you and will support you every step of the way! ❁

Sweet Corn Soup with Cilantro

When the corn is sweet and fresh in the summer, don't miss making this simple soup, which showcases it so beautifully. I like to garnish the soup with a little lime juice and cilantro, but if you prefer to forgo the lime and use another fresh herb, go for it.

Serves 4

For the soup:
8 ears sweet corn (about 20 ounces), shucked
2 teaspoons extra-virgin olive oil
1 medium red onion, cut into medium dice
4 cloves garlic, minced
2 cups low-sodium chicken stock or water
2 cups buttermilk
Salt

For the garnish:
2 limes, cut in half
¼ cup chopped cilantro leaves

METHOD Cut the corn kernels from the cobs, reserving the kernels and cobs separately. Preheat a large Dutch oven or soup kettle over medium heat. Add the oil and onion and cook over medium heat for 4 to 5 minutes or until the onions are translucent. Stir in the corn kernels and cook for 3 minutes. Add the garlic and cook for 2 minutes or until the garlic is fragrant. Add the stock, buttermilk, and reserved corn cobs and simmer, uncovered, for 20 minutes or until the corn is very tender. (Don't be alarmed if the milk solids from the buttermilk rise to the surface of the soup; these will be incorporated when the soup is pureed.)

Remove and discard the corn cobs and puree the soup in a blender or food processor until smooth. Season with salt.

ASSEMBLY Divide the soup among 4 serving bowls. Squeeze lime juice over each bowl and sprinkle with the chopped cilantro.

Per serving: 355 calories • 8 g fat • 2 g sat fat • 5 mg chol • 5 mg sodium • 67 g carb • 17 g sugar • 8 g fiber • 16 g protein • 168 mg calcium

Curried Cauliflower Soup

Cauliflower is a cruciferous vegetable that is too often overlooked in American cooking. Next time you're at the market, pick up a head or two and try this lovely pureed soup lightly seasoned with curry and cumin. Cauliflower is also great roasted and drizzled with just a little extra-virgin olive oil.

Serves 8

For the soup:
2 tablespoons extra-virgin olive oil
2 yellow onions, cut into medium dice
2 teaspoons curry powder
1 teaspoon ground cumin
1 head cauliflower (about 2 pounds), cut into 1-inch florets
6 cups low-sodium chicken stock or vegetable stock
Salt and freshly ground black pepper

For the garnish:
4 teaspoons extra-virgin olive oil
1 lemon, quartered
4 tablespoons chopped chives

METHOD Heat the oil over medium heat in a large Dutch oven or heavy soup pot. Add the onion and cook over medium-high heat, stirring occasionally, for 7 to 10 minutes or until the onion is golden brown. Add the curry powder and cumin to the pot and cook while stirring for 2 minutes or until fragrant.

Add the cauliflower and stock to the pan and bring to a boil. Reduce the heat to a simmer and cover, leaving the lid slightly ajar. Simmer the soup for 30 to 40 minutes or until the cauliflower is very tender.

Using a handheld immersion blender, puree the soup in the pot until it is smooth, or puree it in a food processor. Season the soup with salt and pepper.

ASSEMBLY Divide the soup among 8 serving bowls and drizzle ½ teaspoon olive oil around the top of each bowl. Squeeze a quarter lemon over the soup and sprinkle with the chopped chives.

Per serving: 124 calories • 7 g fat • 1 g sat fat • 0 mg chol • 88 mg sodium • 12 g carb • 5 g sugar • 4 g fiber • 6 g protein • 44 mg calcium

Carb Smart

Nothing I have encountered in the past few years has been more eye opening than what I call "carb confusion." A lot of diets suggest cutting back drastically on carbs and concentrating on protein. This appeals to a lot of people. Who wouldn't rather eat a bacon cheeseburger (without the bun, of course) than a bowl of broccoli? While this approach produces quick weight loss for lots of folks, the pounds return pretty quickly, too.

It turns out it's not so much the amount of carbs you ingest but the *type* of carbs. White bread, sugary soft drinks, sweetened processed cereals, and white pasta are absorbed quickly and thus can cause spikes in blood sugar levels. Not good at all! This can lead to type 2 diabetes, heart disease, and—guess what?—weight gain.

Research shows that whole grains, whole fruits, and vegetables are your best bet for carbs when it comes to good health. Whole wheat bread and pasta, brown rice, and legumes take longer to digest and therefore are better for maintaining steady blood sugar levels. They also leave you feeling satisfied far longer than those "other" carbohydrates. In fact, the Harvard School of Public Health ran a study that showed that those who ate a diet rich in whole grains and other whole foods gained less weight than others over a twenty-year period.

Nothing confusing about that! ❉

$\mathcal{M}$iso Corn Chowder

I love corn chowder in any form, especially during the summer, when the corn is at its best. A few tablespoons of miso transports the chowder to another level. If you want to make this a fuller meal, add some steamed clams.

Serves 4

For the chowder:
1 tablespoon extra-virgin olive oil
1 large yellow onion, cut into small dice
2 cloves garlic, minced
2 tablespoons yellow or red miso paste
3 cups sweet corn kernels
2 stalks celery, peeled and cut into small dice
1 large Yukon Gold potato, peeled and cut into small dice
3 cups low-sodium chicken stock
1 cup buttermilk
Salt and freshly ground black pepper

For the garnish:
8 teaspoons chopped chives

METHOD Heat the oil over medium heat in a large Dutch oven or heavy soup pot. Add the onion and cook over medium heat, stirring occasionally, for 5 minutes or until the onions are translucent. Add the garlic and miso to the pot and cook for 2 more minutes or until fragrant. Add the corn, celery, and potato to the pot. Cook the vegetables for 10 minutes while stirring. Add the stock and bring to a simmer. Continue to simmer for 15 minutes or until the potatoes are tender. Reduce the heat to low and add the buttermilk; do not let it boil. Season the chowder with salt and pepper.

ASSEMBLY Divide the chowder among 4 serving bowls and sprinkle with the chives.

Per serving: 284 calories • 7 g fat • 1 g sat fat • 2 mg chol • 485 mg sodium • 50 g carb • 11 g sugar • 7 g fiber • 11 g protein • 110 mg calcium

Roasted Sweet Potato and Ginger Soup

There are some flavors that beg to be paired, and sweet potatoes and ginger are in that category. This smooth, pureed soup is rich and comforting, ideal for fall evenings.

Serves 6

For the soup:
2 medium sweet potatoes
2 tablespoons extra-virgin olive oil
1 medium yellow onion, cut into small dice
2 tablespoons minced fresh ginger
1 jalapeno pepper, seeded and minced
2 teaspoons ground coriander
½ teaspoon ground nutmeg
4 cups low-sodium chicken stock or water
Salt

For the garnish:
2 green onions, root ends removed, finely chopped

METHOD Preheat the oven to 450°F.

Poke the sweet potatoes with a fork, wrap in aluminum foil, and bake in the oven for 1 hour. Remove from the oven and let cool to room temperature. Cut the sweet potatoes in half and scrape out the flesh.

Heat the oil over medium heat in a large Dutch oven or heavy soup pot. Add the onions and ginger, and cook over medium heat, stirring occasionally, for 5 minutes or until the onions are translucent. Add the jalapeno, coriander, and nutmeg and cook for 3 minutes or until fragrant. Add the roasted sweet potato flesh and stock to the pot. Simmer for 10 minutes. Remove from the heat and puree with a handheld immersion blender or food processor until smooth. Season with salt.

ASSEMBLY Divide the soup among 6 serving bowls and sprinkle with the green onions.

Per serving: 111 calories • 6 g fat • 1 g sat fat • 0 mg chol • 73 mg sodium • 12 g carb • 4 g sugar • 2 g fiber • 4 g protein • 22 mg calcium

Frogmore Stew

~~~~~~

At my Chicago restaurant, TABLE Fifty-Two, we specialize in southern cooking, and this stew is a specialty of South Carolina's Low Country. I don't know why it's called Frogmore Stew, because frogs have nothing to do with it. Instead, it's a comingling of sausage, corn, and shrimp that is usually served at large family gatherings, church suppers, and the like. The shrimp is not peeled, which makes Frogmore Stew one of those "hands-on" dishes where the diners do some of the work and don't worry about the mess. This version is lighter than the restaurant fare but just as tasty!

Serves 6

For the stew:
Juice of 1 lemon
1 pound smoked turkey andouille sausage links
4 ears sweet corn, shucked and broken into 3-inch pieces
3 tablespoons Old Bay seasoning
1 tablespoon red chili flakes
18 medium shrimp in the shell
Salt

For the garnish:
1 lemon, cut into 6 wedges

METHOD In a large stock pot, bring 1 gallon water to a boil. Add the lemon juice, sausage links, corn, Old Bay seasoning, and chili flakes. Reduce to a simmer and cook for 7 minutes. Add the shrimp and cook for an additional 5 minutes or until the shrimp is just cooked. Remove from the heat and drain immediately. Cut the sausage links into 1-inch pieces on the bias. Season with salt.

ASSEMBLY Arrange the Frogmore Stew on a large serving platter, garnish with the lemon wedges, and serve immediately.

Per serving: 240 calories • 9 g fat • 2 g sat fat • 94 mg chol • 877 mg sodium • 24 g carb • 5 g sugar • 3 g fiber • 18 g protein • 10 mg calcium

Lentil and Escarole Soup
with Manchego Cheese

Lentils make a wonderful soup. They go down easily and fill you up like other legumes do. This simple soup is made extra special with a grating of Manchego cheese, a Spanish sheep cheese that is nearly as firm as parmesan. I love the slightly sour flavor of the cheese.

Serves 4

For the soup:
1 tablespoon extra-virgin olive oil
½ medium onion, finely chopped
1 small clove garlic, finely chopped
1 small carrot, coarsely chopped
¾ cup French green lentils
1 18-ounce jar or can tomatoes, drained and coarsely chopped
1 bay leaf
½ bunch escarole, cut crosswise into 1-inch strips (about 3 ounces
    when trimmed and cut)
Salt and freshly ground black pepper

For the garnish:
4 tablespoons grated Manchego cheese
Grated zest of 1 lemon
2 teaspoons extra-virgin olive oil

METHOD Heat the oil over medium heat in a large Dutch oven or heavy soup pot. Add the onion and cook over medium heat, stirring occasionally, for 5 minutes or until the onions are translucent. Add the garlic and carrot and cook until tender, about 3 minutes. Add the lentils, tomatoes, bay leaf, and 5 cups of water. Bring to a boil, reduce heat, and simmer until the lentils are tender, about 40 minutes.

Add the escarole to the soup and cook for 5 minutes more. Season to taste with salt and pepper.

ASSEMBLY Divide the soup among 4 serving bowls and sprinkle with the Manchego cheese and lemon zest to taste, then drizzle with the olive oil.

Per serving: 222 calories • 8 g fat • 2 g sat fat • 5 mg chol • 324 mg sodium • 28 g carb • 5 g sugar • 8 g fiber • 11 g protein • 131 mg calcium

For some reason not everyone embraces the simple lentil. I adore them whether they are of the green, yellow, black, or red variety. Different types of lentils take different amounts of time to cook properly, but once that little lentil is cooked just done, it sings with texture and flavor. I like to refer to lentils as vegetable caviar. Leftover lentils or even over-cooked lentils puree easily in the blender and can be added to the soup.

Jambalaya

New Orleans has produced some of our country's best dishes, and jambalaya is a stellar example of the creative fare to come out of that graceful, old city. Like so many stews, variations are numerous, although jambalaya nearly always includes sausage and seafood (usually shrimp). I have lightened it up, but there's no sacrifice of flavor.

Serves 8

For the jambalaya:
2 teaspoons extra-virgin olive oil
1 pound boneless and skinless chicken thighs, cut into 1-inch pieces
1 pound turkey andouille sausage, sliced
1 large yellow onion, chopped
1 green bell pepper, seeded and chopped
3 cloves garlic, minced
2 stalks celery, peeled and chopped
1 18-ounce jar or can chopped tomatoes
5 cups low-sodium chicken stock or water
1 tablespoon smoked paprika
1 teaspoon garlic powder
1 teaspoon onion powder
1 teaspoon cayenne
2 bay leaves
1 tablespoon hot sauce
1 cup long grain brown rice
Salt and pepper to taste
1 pound large shrimp, peeled and deveined

For the garnish:
¼ cup chopped flat-leaf parsley
¼ cup chopped chives
2 limes, quartered
Hot sauce (optional)

METHOD Place the olive oil in a preheated large Dutch oven or a large pot over medium heat. When the oil is hot, add the chicken and sausage and cook for about 5 minutes, stirring occasionally with a wooden spoon. Then add the onion, bell pepper, garlic, and celery. Cook for 10 minutes or until they begin to soften and become fragrant.

Add the tomatoes, chicken broth, paprika, garlic powder, onion powder, and cayenne to the pot and bring to a simmer. Add the bay leaves and hot sauce, stir in the rice, and season with salt and pepper. Reduce to a low simmer and cover. Cook for 35 minutes or until the rice is about three-quarters done. Add the shrimp to the pot and continue to cook, uncovered, for 10 more minutes or until the shrimp are just cooked. Remove the pot from the heat and let the jambalaya sit, covered, for 30 minutes before serving. During this time, it will thicken a little.

ASSEMBLY Divide the jambalaya among 8 serving bowls and garnish with the chopped parsley and chives (you can mix them together first if you want) and squeezes of lime juice. Season with hot sauce if desired.

Per serving: 388 calories • 13 g fat • 3 g sat fat • 183 mg chol • 920 mg sodium • 30 g carb • 5 g sugar • 3 g fiber • 36 g protein • 71 mg calcium

6

Salads

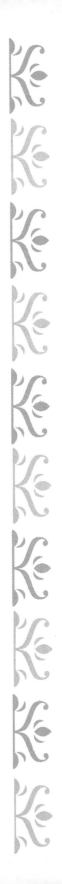

What better way to eat your vegetables than in a salad? There is something pure about salads, whether they are side salads or main courses. I grew up on a farm in Florida where we had a large vegetable garden and a long growing season, and so salads seem both familiar and friendly to me. In the spring when the lettuces were tender and fresh, green salads ruled the table. As the heat built, we ate tomato and cucumber salads. Bean and corn salads found their way onto the table and were great treats. Potato and macaroni salads were as common as grits and fried chicken. Mostly they were made with mayonnaise-based dressings and while I love them this way, these days I tend to use lighter dressings to moisten them if I indulge at all.

Since those childhood days, I have eaten many salads with ingredients I would not have recognized back then: quinoa, feta cheese, pine nuts, and mesclun greens. All are tasty, and all meet the requirement that a salad be a medley of tastes and textures. And like most things in the world of healthy eating, the key to a successful salad is that the ingredients be fresh, fresh, fresh.

Salads are an important part of a healthful diet. If you incorporate a salad into your daily routine, I promise you will feel better. Eating leafy vegetables regularly is better than and just as effective as enduring a three-day liquid "cleanse." If you're feeling listless, a salad a day will change your life. And I am talking to men as well as women. Too many guys seem to think that "real men don't eat salads," which is nonsense and yet prevails. I was eating in a corporate cafeteria a little while ago and noted that the men lined up for burgers, while the women swarmed around the salad bar. Everyone, men and women, should eat salad. And salads can be as filling as any other dish. Try the Curried Chicken Salad with Whole Wheat Pita on page 80 or the Grilled Flank Steak with Red Onions, Tomatoes, and Spinach on page 74. Nothing sissy about these!

I don't mean just any ol' salad. Take care when assembling yours. Stay away from croutons, excessive amounts of cheese, and sweet bottled dressings. This goes for salads from salad bars and restaurants as well as those you make at home. Avoid side salads dressed with mayonnaise or large amounts of oil. When you eat out, always ask for your dressing on the side and use it sparingly; if the greens are fresh and full of life, they taste pretty darn good without the dressing. I have found that lots of folks will eat chopped veggies in a salad when they might not be too keen on those same vegetables served as a side dish. Go figure. The Chopped Salad with Lemon Dressing on page 84 is always a big hit. Try it! Heck, try them all! You will never regret making salad part of your daily life.

Chilled Peas with Heart of Palm, Basil, and Yogurt ✳ 70

Fresh Fennel and Arugula with Meyer Lemon Dressing ✳ 72

Purple Cabbage and Carrot Slaw with Coriander ✳ 73

Grilled Flank Steak Salad with Red Onions, Tomatoes, and Spinach ✳ 74

Chicken and Apples with Blue Cheese–Yogurt Dressing ✳ 76

Chilled Quinoa with Smoked Turkey and Edamame ✳ 78

Curried Chicken Salad with Whole Wheat Pita ✳ 80

Garden Greens with Buttermilk Dressing ✳ 82

Chopped Salad with Lemon Dressing ✳ 84

Warm Kale and Summer Squash with Ricotta Salata ✳ 86

Watermelon and Feta with Lime and Serrano Chili Peppers ✳ 88

Cucumber with Mint and Pomegranate Seeds ✳ 89

Shaved Brussels Sprout Salad with Pine Nuts and Lemon ✳ 90

Chilled Peas with Heart of Palm, Basil, and Yogurt

~~~~~~

In this sumptuous little salad, peas flavored with a creamy yogurt dressing nestle next to a tangy salad made from heart of palm. Each is better than the other and both taste perfect together. I like heart of palm because it is high in fiber and protein and low in cholesterol. It is harvested from the trunks of palm trees, as you might suspect from the name, and if you can't find it for this recipe, use canned artichoke hearts packed in water or a simple brine.

Serves 4

For the peas:
¼ cup nonfat Greek yogurt
2 tablespoons extra-virgin olive oil
1 tablespoon lemon juice
3 cups shucked peas, blanched and chilled
Salt and freshly ground black pepper

For the heart of palm:
4 stalks heart of palm
1 tablespoon extra-virgin olive oil
2 teaspoons lemon juice
Salt and freshly ground pepper

For the garnish:
8 leaves Bibb lettuce, washed
8 leaves fresh basil, chopped

METHOD **To prepare the peas:** In a medium mixing bowl, whisk together the yogurt, oil, and lemon juice until thoroughly combined. Gently fold the peas into the yogurt mixture and season with salt and pepper.

To prepare the heart of palm: Slice the heart of palm into ¼-inch-thick rings on the bias and place in a small mixing bowl. Add the olive oil and lemon juice and toss until combined. Season to taste with salt and pepper.

ASSEMBLY Place two leaves of the Bibb lettuce on each plate. Spoon some of the pea mixture and heart of palm into each lettuce piece. Sprinkle the chopped basil over the peas and heart of palm. Serve immediately.

Per serving: 189 calories • 11 g fat • 2 g sat fat • 0 mg chol • 147 mg sodium • 16 g carb • 1 g sugar • 5 g fiber • 8 g protein • 36 mg calcium

Stand Up!

I've said it before and will say it again: you can't lose weight without exercising. But before you shake your head in dismay, wait! You don't have to hit the gym day after day or put on your running shoes for a few laps around the neighborhood. Just moving more than usual helps a lot.

Cutting back on the amount of time you sit around is as crucial as increasing the amount of time you exercise. Long periods of inactivity can alter your metabolism and make it more difficult to lose weight. Plus you are more apt to suffer from heart disease, hypertension, type 2 diabetes, and other health problems related to obesity.

So, if you are one of those Americans who sit for hours and hours at the office, in the car, or just planted on the sofa with the television blaring, make a change. Stand up! Walk around the room, up and down the stairs—or, better yet, go for a brisk walk that lasts for at least twenty minutes. Before you know it, you'll be walking for thirty minutes, forty minutes, fifty minutes . . . ❉

Fresh Fennel and Arugula with Meyer Lemon Dressing

~~~~~~

I love crunchy fennel and peppery arugula dressed with a slightly sweet dressing made from Meyer lemons—a fresh-tasting pick-me-up. Meyer lemons are only available in the wintertime, so if you can't find them, use regular lemon juice and replace a third of it with fresh orange juice.

Serves 4

For the dressing:
6 tablespoons extra-virgin olive oil
3 tablespoons Meyer lemon juice
Salt and freshly ground black pepper

For the salad:
2 medium fennel bulbs
2 oranges, peeled and separated into segments
4 cups baby arugula leaves

METHOD To prepare the dressing: Place the olive oil and lemon juice in a small glass jar with a lid and season with salt and pepper. Secure the lid and shake until thoroughly combined. Refrigerate until ready to use.

To prepare the salad: Remove the green, feathery stalks from the fennel bulb, thinly slice the white part of the fennel bulb on a Japanese mandoline or with a knife. The thinner you cut the fennel the better. Place the sliced fennel in a medium mixing bowl and toss with 2 tablespoons of the prepared dressing. Let sit for 30 minutes (this will soften the fennel slices a bit). Add the orange segments to the bowl and toss gently.

Place the arugula in a medium mixing bowl and toss with remaining dressing.

ASSEMBLY Divide the arugula among 4 plates and top with some of the fennel mixture. Season with a twist of freshly ground black pepper.

Per serving: 255 calories • 21 g fat • 3 g sat fat • 0 mg chol • 66 mg sodium • 18 g carb • 7 g sugar • 6 g fiber • 3 g protein • 116 mg calcium

$\mathscr{P}$urple Cabbage and Carrot Slaw with Coriander

If you, like me, have come to prefer coleslaws made with oil and vinegar to the more traditional mayonnaise-based varieties, you will love this one! It's chock full of great textures and tastes, including golden raisins, fresh ginger, fiery jalapeno, and fresh lime juice.

Serves 4

¾ cup golden raisins
½ small- to medium-head purple cabbage
2 large carrots, peeled
1 jalapeno pepper, seeded and minced
1 teaspoon minced fresh ginger
1 teaspoon stevia
¼ cup fresh lime juice
3 tablespoons extra-virgin olive oil
3 tablespoons red wine vinegar
1 tablespoon coriander seeds, toasted
Salt and freshly ground black pepper
½ cup chopped cilantro

METHOD Put the raisins in a small bowl and cover with warm water. Set aside to soak for about 10 minutes. Finely shred the purple cabbage in a food processor or with a large, sharp knife and place in a large mixing bowl. Grate the carrot using a box grater and add to the cabbage. Drain the raisins and add them to the slaw with the jalapeno, ginger, stevia, lime juice, olive oil, red wine vinegar, and coriander seeds. Mix until thoroughly combined. Season with salt and pepper. Cover with plastic wrap and refrigerate for 1 hour. Just prior to serving, fold in the cilantro.

ASSEMBLY Divide the slaw equally among 4 serving bowls and enjoy.

Per serving: 297 calories • 14 g fat • 2 g sat fat • 0 mg chol • 75 mg sodium • 41 g carb • 31 g sugar • 8 g fiber • 4 g protein • 122 mg calcium

Grilled Flank Steak Salad with Red Onions, Tomatoes, and Spinach

Most folks like a good steak salad in the summer. I know I do. You can grill the steak and onions a little before dinnertime and keep them warm under foil so you don't have to bother with them when your guests arrive or the family assembles. Both taste great with summer's best tomatoes, too.

Serves 4

For the dressing:
6 tablespoons extra-virgin olive oil
2 tablespoons balsamic vinegar
2 tablespoons chopped fresh basil
Salt and freshly ground black pepper

For the steak and onions:
20 ounces flank steak
1 red onion, peeled and sliced ½ inch thick

For the salad:
4 medium tomatoes, cut into eighths
8 cups baby spinach, cleaned with thick stems discarded
Salt and freshly ground black pepper

METHOD To prepare the dressing: In a medium mason jar with a lid, mix together the olive oil, vinegar, and basil, then season with salt and pepper. Secure the lid and shake until combined (the dressing may separate when it sits, but you can quickly shake it again to combine the ingredients if needed).

To prepare the steak and onions: Preheat a grill to moderate heat.

Rub the steak and onions with 2 tablespoons of the dressing. Place the steak and onions on the grill over moderate heat. Cook the steak for 7 minutes on each side or until medium rare. Cook the onions for 5 minutes on each side or until caramelized. Remove the steak and onions from the grill.

Chop the onions into bite-size pieces. Let the steak rest for 5 minutes, then slice across the grain into ¼-inch-thick slices.

To prepare the salad: In a large mixing bowl, combine the tomatoes, spinach, and grilled red onion. Toss with the remaining dressing. Season with salt and pepper.

ASSEMBLY Divide the salad among 4 serving plates and top each serving with sliced flank steak.

Per serving: 460 calories • 29 g fat • 6 g sat fat • 52 mg chol • 153 mg sodium • 19 g carb • 9 g sugar • 6 g fiber • 33 g protein • 89 mg calcium

Chicken and Apples with
Blue Cheese–Yogurt Dressing

I have never met a chicken salad I didn't like, and this is one of my favorites. I lightened it up by using yogurt instead of mayonnaise, and I toss the tender chicken with apples, apricots, and red onion. The blue cheese pulls everything together.

Serves 4

For the dressing:
¼ cup nonfat Greek yogurt
1 tablespoon extra-virgin olive oil
1 tablespoon lemon juice
¼ cup crumbled blue cheese
2 tablespoons chopped chives
Freshly ground black pepper

For the chicken:
2 skinless and boneless chicken breasts
2 cups buttermilk
1 Granny Smith apple, thinly sliced
¼ cup chopped dried apricots
¼ cup thinly sliced red onion
1 celery stalk, peeled and sliced thin on the bias
Juice of 1 lemon
Salt

METHOD **To prepare the dressing:** In a medium mixing bowl, combine the Greek yogurt, olive oil, and lemon juice. Stir with a wooden spoon until all the ingredients are incorporated. Fold in the blue cheese and chives and season with freshly ground black pepper. Refrigerate the dressing until ready to use. (This dressing can be made 3 days in advance.)

To prepare the chicken: Place the chicken breasts and buttermilk in a medium sauté pan and bring to a simmer. The buttermilk will appear to curdle or break—this is okay, as the milk will be discarded once the chicken is cooked. Simmer the chicken in the milk for 20 minutes or until the chicken is just cooked through. Remove from heat and lift the chicken from the buttermilk. Refrigerate the chicken for 30 minutes.

Cut the chicken into bite-size pieces and place in a large mixing bowl. Add the apple, dried apricots, red onion, celery, and lemon juice to the bowl and mix together until combined. Fold in the dressing until fully incorporated and season with salt if desired.

ASSEMBLY Divide the chicken salad among 4 plates.

Per serving: 241 calories • 9 g fat • 3 g sat fat • 48 mg chol • 300 mg sodium • 21 g carb • 17 g sugar • 2 g fiber • 21 g protein • 219 mg calcium

Chilled Quinoa with Smoked Turkey and Edamame

~~~~~~

Grain salads are delicious any time of year, although I tend to gravitate to them in the summer and fall. Quinoa (KEEN-wah), an ancient grain that has experienced a joyful renaissance in the last decade or so, is one of my favorites. These days I eat it regularly, and always happily. (I call it a grain because it behaves like one, although officially it's a seed.) Quinoa is a perfect protein, cooks in less than half an hour, and tastes nutty and pleasingly crunchy. Here I mix it with smoked turkey and shelled fresh soybeans, also known as edamame, for a bold, filling main course salad.

Serves 4

1 cup quinoa, rinsed
½ pound smoked turkey, cubed (about 1½ cups)
1 cup shelled soybeans (also called edamame)
¼ cup chopped flat-leaf parsley
4 green onions, chopped
1 medium tomato, chopped
3 tablespoons lemon juice
2 tablespoons extra-virgin olive oil
Salt and freshly ground black pepper

METHOD Place the quinoa in a medium saucepan and cover with 2 cups cold water. Bring to a boil and immediately reduce to a simmer. Cover with the lid slightly ajar and continue to cook over low heat for 15 to 20 minutes or until the quinoa is puffed and you see a little white ring release from around the quinoa. Remove from the heat and let cool to room temperature.

Place the cooked quinoa in a large mixing bowl and add the smoked turkey, soybeans, parsley, green onions, tomato, lemon juice, and olive oil. Mix together with a wooden spoon until thoroughly combined. Season with salt and pepper.

ASSEMBLY Divide the quinoa salad among 4 plates. This salad can be served at room temperature or chilled.

Per serving: 326 calories • 13 g fat • 2 g sat fat • 26 mg chol • 504 mg sodium • 36 g carb • 3 g sugar • 5 g fiber • 20 g protein • 58 mg calcium

Find Your Happy

Losing weight is a long and potholed road. You can't decide one morning to cut back on soda and pretzels, expecting that a week later your jeans will fit like a dream. Instead, it's a day-in, day-out commitment, while the rest of your life keeps humming along.

This reality makes losing weight a solitary endeavor. Sure, your friends and family members may compliment you on a few lost pounds, but they are just as likely to encourage you to have that margarita after work or join them for a pizza and a movie. You and you alone decide which social events to embrace and which to avoid, what to eat and what to bypass, when to exercise and for how long—and part of doing so means finding what I call "your happy."

What makes you feel good? What signals success? I looked at the folks who surrounded me every day and discovered that some of the most supportive were not those I expected. People I didn't know too well became my Rock of Gibraltar, while some of my closest buddies were threatened by my need to take charge of my girth. Some people are intimidated by change. They thought that because I was making big changes, they should, too—and they didn't want to. A few people even dismissed my efforts as a midlife crisis.

Despite this small number of naysayers, I encountered a large group of encouraging people. Those who sustained me were a surprising lot, and this made me happy.

For example, the chefs at the restaurants cooked very carefully for me—and made sure I drank a lot of water. My friend Kenneth Robling created hour-long music mixes for my iPod to keep me rockin' while I worked out. Others, both close friends and casual acquaintances, never forgot to ask about my efforts and to cheer me on from the sidelines. I learned to steer clear of negative people and instead hang out with those who showed positive energy.

My happy kept me on track and focused on the task before me. I kept optimistic thoughts in my head, chose wisely when I needed someone to talk to, and came to look forward to my daily workouts. Without this happy place, I am not sure I would have made it. But I did! ❄

Curried Chicken Salad with Whole Wheat Pita

~~~~~~

Curry and chicken go together like love and marriage, and just like love, it's a subject I never tire of. I can't think of a better chicken curry salad than this one. When served in whole wheat pita pockets, this makes a perfect lunch or light supper.

Serves 4

For the chicken:
2 boneless, skinless chicken breasts
2 teaspoons extra-virgin olive oil
1 tablespoon yellow curry paste
½ cup nonfat Greek yogurt
2 tablespoons lemon juice
1 green bell pepper, seeded and cut into small dice
⅓ cup coarsely chopped cashews
Salt and freshly ground black pepper

For the garnish:
2 whole wheat pitas, cut in half
2 green onions, thinly sliced

METHOD Preheat the oven to 425°F.

Place the chicken breasts on a nonstick baking sheet. Rub the tops with the olive oil and 1 teaspoon of the yellow curry paste. Bake for 20 minutes or until the chicken is just cooked. Remove from the oven and cool the chicken to room temperature. Shred the chicken into bite-size pieces and place in a large mixing bowl.

In a small bowl, combine the remaining 2 teaspoons of yellow curry paste, the yogurt, and the lemon juice. Mix until fully combined.

Add the yogurt mixture, bell pepper, and cashews to the mixing bowl with the chicken. Toss together until fully incorporated. Season with salt and pepper. Refrigerate for 1 hour.

ASSEMBLY Place a piece of the pita on each plate. Spoon equal amounts of the curried chicken salad inside the pita and sprinkle the green onion over the salad. Top with freshly ground black pepper.

Per serving: 224 calories • 10 g fat • 2 g sat fat • 37 mg chol • 122 mg sodium • 16 g carb • 3 g sugar • 3 g fiber • 20 g protein • 49 mg calcium

This recipe works great with grilled, poached, or baked chicken. I love spooning into lettuce leaves and rolling them up as a snack. I love the aromas of curry in this recipe; it reminds me of getting lost (on purpose) in the spice markets of Singapore. But if curry is not your thing, try smoky paprika or mustard.

Garden Greens with Buttermilk Dressing

As a rule, I stay clear of creamy dressings, preferring to get my calories elsewhere, but because every now and then I feel like indulging, I couldn't resist developing a "healthy" creamy dressing. Prepared with irresistible Greek yogurt and buttermilk made zippy with vinegar and lemon juice, this is not especially thick, but it is gorgeously creamy. Spoon this over your favorite mixed greens and enjoy a glorious side salad.

Serves 8

For the buttermilk dressing:
½ cup nonfat Greek yogurt
½ cup buttermilk
4 tablespoons extra-virgin olive oil
2 tablespoons grainy mustard
2 tablespoons chopped capers
1 tablespoon red wine vinegar
1 tablespoon fresh lemon juice
1 shallot, minced
2 teaspoons chopped fresh oregano
1 tablespoon chopped fresh basil
½ teaspoon stevia
4 dashes hot sauce
Salt and freshly ground black pepper

For the salad:
16 cups mixed salad greens, cleaned
1 cucumber, thinly sliced
1 pint grape tomatoes, cut in half
8 radishes, thinly sliced

METHOD To prepare the dressing: In a mason jar with a lid, combine the yogurt, buttermilk, olive oil, mustard, capers, vinegar, lemon juice, shallot, oregano, basil, stevia, and hot sauce. Shake well to blend. Season with salt and pepper. Refrigerate until ready to use. The dressing can be kept for up to one week in the refrigerator.

To prepare the salad: Place the salad greens, cucumber, tomatoes, and radishes in a large mixing bowl and toss with the buttermilk dressing.

ASSEMBLY Divide the salad among 8 chilled salad plates and top with freshly ground black pepper.

Per serving: 109 calories • 7 g fat • 1 g sat fat • 1 mg chol • 180 mg sodium • 10 g carb • 6 g sugar • 4 g fiber • 4 g protein • 44 mg calcium

I can't say enough about having a great dressing already made in your refrigerator. It really helps me reach for a bowl of salad or some sliced vegetables when that after-noon snack attack comes on. Substituting Greek yogurt for the mayonnaise that is traditionally used in buttermilk dressing is one of the simplest flavor-satisfying changes that I have made to date in my kitchen. It is a win win!

Chopped Salad with Lemon Dressing

Were you to run across me at Southern Art, the restaurant I own in Atlanta, chances are I'd be eating this fantastic chopped salad. I have always liked chopped salads, but I had no idea how popular this would be when we put it on the menu. Everyone loves it! When I feel like making it a full-blown meal, I ask the cooks to grill some shrimp or chicken to eat with it.

Serves 4

For the lemon dressing:
3 tablespoons fresh lemon juice
1 teaspoon honey
1 tablespoon Dijon mustard
2 teaspoons unfiltered apple cider vinegar
2 tablespoons chopped flat-leaf parsley
1 tablespoon chopped fresh tarragon
½ cup extra-virgin olive oil
Salt and freshly ground black pepper

For the salad:
1 head radicchio lettuce
8 leaves romaine lettuce
1 cup grated carrot
1 cup diced cucumber
1 cup diced tomato
¼ cup chopped peanuts
2 hard-cooked eggs, chopped
12 seedless red grapes, quartered
4 radishes, thinly sliced
½ cup crumbled blue cheese

METHOD To prepare the dressing: Place the lemon juice, honey, Dijon mustard, vinegar, parsley, tarragon, and olive oil in a mason jar with a lid. Secure the lid and shake until fully incorporated. Season with salt and pepper.

To prepare the salad: Cut the head of radicchio in half and finely chop into thin strands. Lay the romaine lettuce leaves on top of one another and finely chop them into thin strands. Place the lettuces in a large mixing bowl. Add the carrot, cucumber, tomato, peanuts, eggs, red grapes, radishes, and blue cheese to the mixing bowl. Toss all the ingredients together until fully incorporated.

ASSEMBLY Just prior to serving, toss the salad with the Lemon Dressing. Divide the salad among 4 serving plates and top with freshly ground black pepper.

Per serving: 450 calories • 40 g fat • 9 g sat fat • 119 mg chol • 387 mg sodium • 16 g carb • 8 g sugar • 4 g fiber • 11 g protein • 152 mg calcium

Warm Kale and Summer Squash
with Ricotta Salata

~~~~~~~~~~~~~~~~~~~~~~~~~~~~~~~~~~~~~~~

The flavors and textures of kale and summer squash complement each other perfectly, one bold and crunchy and the other mild and soft. I came up with this warm salad to showcase these two favorites and set them off with shaved ricotta salata. What's ricotta salata? It's aged, semifirm ricotta with a crumbly texture.

Serves 4

For the kale and summer squash:
12 kale leaves, rinsed
2 tablespoons extra-virgin olive oil
1 large shallot, minced
2 summer squash, cut into ¼-inch-thick pieces
1 tablespoon balsamic vinegar
Salt and freshly ground black pepper

For the garnish:
¼ cup pepitos (pumpkin seeds)
½ cup shaved ricotta salata

METHOD Cut the kale leaves from their thick stems and tear into 1-inch-wide pieces. Heat the olive oil in a large sauté pan over medium heat. Add the shallots and cook over medium heat for 2 minutes or until translucent. Add the summer squash to the pan and cook over medium-high heat for 7 minutes or until the squash begins to caramelize. Add the kale to the pan and cover. Cook for 2 minutes or until the kale is just wilted. Add the balsamic vinegar to the pan and season with salt and pepper. Remove from the heat.

ASSEMBLY Divide the kale and summer squash among 4 plates and sprinkle the pepitos and shaved ricotta salata over the vegetables. Top with freshly ground black pepper.

Per serving: 190 calories • 14 g fat • 4 g sat fat • 13 mg chol • 254 mg sodium • 11 g carb • 4 g sugar • 2 g fiber • 7 g protein • 74 mg calcium

What Makes an Oil Healthful?

Most people know that extra-virgin olive oil is better for you than most oils. But what about the other oils? Is peanut oil okay? Should you use canola or sunflower oil? Are all olive oils the same?

There is an easy answer, and then a more nuanced one.

Olive oil and canola oil are probably the best choices for cooking and baking. Use olive oil for the former, canola for the latter (although there are recipes where switching this formula makes sense). When you need a high smoke point, turn to canola; for uncooked preparations (salad dressings), grab the olive oil. Nonetheless, Italians readily fry and sauté using the best extra-virgin olive oil they can afford, with delicious results.

That's the easy part of the explanation. What follows is a little more complex.

What you don't want is saturated fat. This is found most commonly in animal products (dairy) and meat. It's also present in small amounts in every fat (oil), although the most guilty are coconut and palm oils.

After shunning saturated fats, you next want to avoid polyunsaturated fats. Polyunsaturated fats are far more acceptable than saturated fats, but the first choice for fat is monounsaturated. Olive oil contains 78 percent monounsaturated fats, 8 percent polyunsaturated, and 14 percent saturated. Canola oil is 62 percent monounsaturated, 31 percent polyunsaturated, and 7 percent saturated.

If you look at those numbers, you might argue that olive oil, with higher levels of saturated fat, is worse than canola oil. But the higher amount of monounsaturated fat counterbalances the saturated fat. In the end, both oils are good choices.

Sunflower oil is another good one, with 79 percent monounsaturated fat. Corn oil, not a terrible choice, is 25 percent monounsaturated and 62 percent polyunsaturated (13 percent saturated).

Recent research indicates that the degree to which an oil is processed is also critical. Extra virgin or virgin olive oil is extracted mechanically—not chemically—from the olives. High-quality fruit, prompt crushing, and minimal processing help maintain the olives' naturally occurring antioxidants, called polyphenols and tocopherols.

Polyphenols are credited with helping guard against cardiovascular disease, osteoporosis, and some cancers. The better the quality of the extra-virgin olive oil, the higher the polyphenol content.

So, what to do? Rely on olive oil, canola oil, and sunflower oil. Use high-quality extra-virgin oils whenever possible, because they are less processed and better for you.

I guess it's not that complicated after all! ❈

Watermelon and Feta with Lime and Serrano Chili Peppers

~~~~~~

Believe it or not, watermelon and feta make a great pairing. Toss in some hot chili peppers and cilantro and you have a salad to delight everyone who tries it. Buy seedless watermelon for this—you won't be disappointed when you try it!

Serves 8

3 pounds seedless watermelon, rind removed, cut into large dice
   (about 6 cups)
2 serrano chili peppers, seeded and minced
Juice of 1 lime
½ cup low-fat feta cheese, crumbled
¼ cup cilantro leaves

METHOD Place the watermelon in a large mixing bowl. Add the minced serrano chili pepper and lime juice to the bowl and toss gently until combined. Sprinkle with the feta and cilantro leaves and toss once more to incorporate. Refrigerate until ready to serve.

Per serving: 54 calories • 1 g fat • 1 g sat fat • 3 mg chol • 119 mg sodium • 9 g carb • 7 g sugar • 1 g fiber • 3 g protein • 34 mg calcium

Cucumber with Mint and Pomegranate Seeds

I am especially fond of these chilled, crisp cucumbers, which I munch on whenever I can. They are just the thing to curb my appetite. Plus, I love how the pomegranate seeds pop in my mouth and fill it with sweet-tart flavor.

Serves 6 to 8

2 cucumbers
2 tablespoons red wine vinegar
2 tablespoons extra-virgin olive oil
1 pomegranate, seeded
2 tablespoons chopped mint
Salt and freshly ground black pepper

METHOD Peel the cucumbers and slice them ¼ inch thick. Place them in a large mixing bowl and add the red wine vinegar, olive oil, pomegranate seeds, and mint. Toss all the ingredients together and season with salt and pepper.

ASSEMBLY Place the cucumbers in a large serving bowl and enjoy immediately.

Per serving: 68 calories • 4 g fat • 1 g sat fat • 0 mg chol • 1 mg sodium • 8 g carb • 6 g sugar • 2 g fiber • 1 g protein • 20 mg calcium

Shaved Brussels Sprout Salad with
Pine Nuts and Lemon

~~~~~~

Don't like brussels sprouts? Let me change your mind with this zesty raw salad. Most people can't believe what they're eating and enjoying so much. If you prefer, substitute feta cheese for the pecorino Romano.

Serves 4

20 medium brussels sprouts, cleaned
4 tablespoons extra-virgin olive oil
2 tablespoons fresh lemon juice
¼ cup pine nuts
¼ cup grated pecorino Romano cheese
Salt and freshly ground black pepper

METHOD Cut the brussels sprouts in half lengthwise. Thinly slice them until you get to the chunky white core of the brussels sprout (about three-fourths of the way down), then discard the rest of the brussels sprout. Place the sliced brussels sprouts in a medium mixing bowl and add the olive oil, lemon juice, pine nuts, and pecorino Romano cheese. Mix thoroughly. Season with salt and pepper. Cover and let sit for 30 minutes to let the flavors marry before serving.

ASSEMBLY Divide the brussels sprout salad among 4 bowls and top with freshly ground black pepper.

Per serving: 250 calories • 22 g fat • 4 g sat fat • 8 mg chol • 151 mg sodium • 10 g carb • 3 g sugar • 4 g fiber • 7 g protein • 132 mg calcium

Vegetarian Main Courses

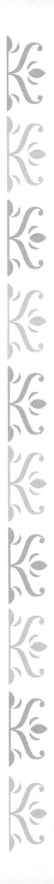

Okay, America. Mom was right. Eat your vegetables. Most of us don't have to reach back to our childhoods to know that vegetables are "good for us." Just as surely as we know that french fries are not the best choice for a snack, we know that we should eat vegetables with every lunch and dinner. It's been my experience that folks who are overweight often don't eat enough veggies, or they fool themselves into thinking that those fast-food fries meet the criteria. Everyone, obese or not, who cares about their health should make a decision to include more vegetables in their daily diets. I have cooked for families who designate at least one day a week as vegetarian. No meat or fish on the menu, just vegetarian main courses that are every bit as satisfying and interesting as any other main course. A good idea for everyone.

I grew up on a farm where it was commonplace to eat meals composed solely of vegetables. It might be a tomato sandwich for lunch (just a dab of mayo and a good sprinkling of salt and pepper), fresh peas and rice, tomatoes cooked with okra, or a squash casserole. We cooked, ate, and enjoyed whatever was in season. Later, I noticed that it was unusual to find vegetarian main courses on restaurant menus. Times have changed, and more and more restaurants offer meatless main courses. Great news. A few years ago, I teamed up with a wonderful guy named Tal Ronnen, a well-known vegan chef who draws on his classical training to create amazing food. We developed the menu for LYFE Kitchen in Palo Alto, California, a coming together of my southern-comfort style and Mr. Vegan Fresh. During that process I fell in love all over again with all sorts of vegetables. I had never strayed far from them, but Tal reminded me of their incredible life force, vibrancy, and diversity. Vegetarian entrees are soul satisfying, and you don't have to be a vegetarian or vegan to enjoy them. You simply have to be someone who likes food and appreciates its health-giving properties. Remember, Mom was right: vegetables are important, and the more the merrier!

Eggplant Parmesan with Garlic Rapini ✳ 93

Whole Grain Griddle Bread with Goat Cheese ✳ 96

Vegetable Shepherd's Pie ✳ 98

Roasted Poblano Tamales ✳ 100

Baked Polenta with Tomato Sauce and Ricotta ✳ 102

Slow-Cooked Farro with Asparagus and Pecorino Cheese ✳ 104

Shirataki Noodles Stir-Fry ✳ 106

Potato Tart with Mustard Greens and Lemon Thyme ✳ 108

Dirty Rice with Mushroom Bolognese ✳ 112

Art Smith's Healthy Comfort

Eggplant Parmesan with Garlic Rapini

~~~~~~

When we put this eggplant parm on the menu at LYFE Kitchen in Palo Alto, California, our customers were ecstatic—a healthful version of an old favorite made with garden-fresh eggplant, garlicky rapini, and one of my favorite tomato sauces. The sauce gets its deep, rich flavor from the whole roasted onion and entire garlic bulb. I rely on this sauce in the recipe for Baked Polenta with Tomato Sauce and Ricotta on page 102 and for Swordfish with Capers, Olives, Tomato Sauce, and Whole Wheat Penne on page 130. Why argue with success?

Serves 4

For the tomato sauce:
4 tomatoes
1 medium yellow onion, skin on
1 small bulb garlic
2 tablespoons extra-virgin olive oil
Salt

For the ricotta:
1 cup ricotta cheese
2 tablespoons chopped fresh basil

For the eggplant:
2 small eggplants
½ cup whole wheat pastry flour
2 large eggs, lightly beaten
1 cup whole wheat panko breadcrumbs
2 tablespoons grated Parmesan cheese
Salt and freshly ground black pepper

For the rapini:
2 tablespoons extra-virgin olive oil
4 cloves garlic, smashed
8 pieces rapini (also called broccoli rabe)
Salt and freshly ground black pepper

For the garnish:
4 tablespoons chopped fresh basil
2 tablespoons grated Parmesan cheese

METHOD To prepare the tomato sauce: Preheat the oven to 425°F.

Place the tomatoes, yellow onion, and garlic in a baking pan. Bake for 45 minutes or until the garlic is soft and the skin is peeling away from the tomatoes. Remove from the oven and cool to room temperature. Remove the skin from the tomatoes and put in a saucepan. Squeeze the garlic pulp from the cloves and add to the tomatoes. Remove and discard the onion's skin and coarsely chop the onion. Add to the tomatoes. Add the olive oil to the tomatoes and puree with a handheld immersion blender or in a blender until smooth. You may need to add up to ⅓ cup of water if there is not enough liquid. Season with salt.

Warm the tomato sauce just prior to use.

To prepare the ricotta: In a small mixing bowl, combine the ricotta cheese and basil. Refrigerate until ready to use.

To prepare the eggplant: Preheat the oven to 425°F.

Slice the eggplants into eight 1-inch-thick pieces. Lightly coat the eggplant pieces with the whole wheat pastry flour, patting off any excess. Place the eggs in a mixing bowl and coat the eggplant slices with the egg. Place the panko and Parmesan cheese in a mixing bowl and season with salt and pepper. After the eggplant has been coated in the egg, immediately coat it in the panko bread crumb mixture.

Place the breaded eggplant pieces on a nonstick baking sheet and bake for 20 minutes or until golden brown and tender.

Remove from the oven and place 1 tablespoon of the ricotta mixture over the eggplant pieces. Return to the oven for 5 minutes to warm the ricotta cheese.

To prepare the rapini: Warm the olive oil in a large sauté pan, add the smashed garlic, and continue to cook over medium heat for 1 minute to infuse the garlic into the oil. Add the rapini to the pan and cook for 7 to 10 minutes or until the rapini is cooked al dente. Season with salt and pepper.

ASSEMBLY Spoon ½ cup of the tomato sauce on each plate and top with two pieces of the eggplant Parmesan. Arrange two pieces of the rapini over the eggplant Parmesan. Sprinkle the basil and Parmesan cheese over the rapini.

Per serving: 455 calories • 24 g fat • 7 g sat fat • 131 mg chol • 218 mg sodium • 46 g carb • 11 g sugar • 12 g fiber • 20 g protein • 314 mg calcium

Whole Grain Griddle Bread with Goat Cheese

~~~~~~

I love this for dinner when I don't feel like a big meal but crave something "homemade" and reassuring. You'll have to plan ahead to make it, but the griddle bread is worth the effort. While you could top it with any number of foods, I chose smooth, creamy goat cheese and basil. These are sort of like minipizzas, only better!

Serves 6

For the griddle bread:
½ package dry yeast
½ cup warm water
2 teaspoons agave syrup
1½ cups 7-grain flour (Great Rivers Organic Milling brand)
½ cup whole wheat pastry flour
½ teaspoon sea salt
½ teaspoon ground coriander
½ teaspoon ground cumin
½ teaspoon baking powder
½ cup soy or almond milk
½ cup nonfat Greek yogurt
2 tablespoons flaxseeds
Cooking spray

For the toppings:
6 tablespoons extra-virgin olive oil
1 cup minced red onion
4 ounces goat cheese (about ½ cup)
1 teaspoon dried red pepper flakes

For the garnish:
6 tablespoons chopped basil

METHOD **To prepare the griddle bread:** Sprinkle the yeast over the warm water, add the agave, and let sit for 10 minutes.

In a large mixing bowl, combine the 7-grain and whole wheat flours, salt, coriander, cumin, and baking powder.

Warm the soy milk over low heat, but do not bring to a simmer (it should just be warm to the touch). Add the yeast mixture to the warm milk.

Make a well in the middle of the flour and add the milk mixture. Mix with your hands until incorporated. Add the yogurt and flaxseeds to the mixture and knead the dough until smooth but still a little sticky. Place in an oiled 1-gallon plastic bag and refrigerate for 3 hours.

Heat a cast iron or nonstick griddle over medium heat.

Divide the dough into 6 even portions. Form each one into a ball and roll out on a lightly floured surface until it is about a 6-inch circle.

Spray the griddle with cooking spray and cook for 3 to 4 minutes on each side or until just cooked. Remove from the pan and repeat with the remaining dough.

To prepare the griddle bread with the toppings: Preheat the oven to 425°F.

Brush each cooked griddle bread with the olive oil and top with the red onion, goat cheese, and red pepper flakes. Place on a baking sheet. Bake for 15 minutes or until the cheese begins to turn golden brown.

ASSEMBLY Cut each griddle bread into 4 pieces, sprinkle with the basil, and place on each serving plate.

Per serving: 385 calories • 21 g fat • 5 g sat fat • 9 mg chol • 9 mg sodium • 38 g carb • 5 g sugar • 6 g fiber • 13 g protein • 91 mg calcium

Vegetable Shepherd's Pie

Classic shepherd's pie made with ground lamb was developed as a way to use up the leftover meat from the Sunday roast. I have moved it squarely off that table and into a new, more modern realm with a tempting mélange of vegetables topped with potatoes mashed with buttermilk and olive oil to make them extra good.

Serves 4

For the potatoes:
1 pound Yukon Gold potatoes, peeled and cut into 1-inch chunks
½ cup buttermilk
2 tablespoons extra-virgin olive oil
Zest of one lemon
Salt and freshly ground black pepper

For the filling:
1 tablespoon extra-virgin olive oil
1 large onion, finely diced
½ cup finely diced carrot
¾ cup corn kernels
1 teaspoon chopped fresh thyme
2 tablespoons whole wheat pastry flour
1 cup vegetable broth
1 15-ounce can black beans, rinsed and drained
2 tablespoons chopped chives or flat-leaf parsley

METHOD To prepare the potatoes: Place the potatoes in a large saucepan and cover with water. Bring to a simmer over medium-high heat, then reduce the heat to medium. Cook for 10 to 15 minutes or until tender. Drain the potatoes and return them to the pot. Add the buttermilk and olive oil and mash with a potato masher until almost smooth. Fold in the lemon zest and season with salt and pepper.

To prepare the filling: Preheat the broiler.

In a large sauté pan, warm the oil over medium-high heat and add the onions. Cook for 7 minutes or until the onions are translucent. Add the carrots to the pan and continue to cook for 5 minutes. Add the corn and thyme and cook for 3 minutes. Add the flour and stir to coat the vegetables. Add the vegetable broth and bring to a simmer. Cook for 1 minute. Add the black beans and cook for 2 more minutes or until hot. Fold in the chopped chives or parsley.

Place the hot vegetables in an 8-inch broiling pan and top with the mashed potatoes. Broil for 6 to 10 minutes or until the potato is lightly browned.

ASSEMBLY Divide the shepherd's pie among 4 serving plates.

Per serving: 341 calories • 12 g fat • 2 g sat fat • 1 mg chol • 495 mg sodium • 51 g carb • 6 g sugar • 9 g fiber • 10 g protein • 104 mg calcium

Roasted Poblano Tamales

In Mexico, tamales are often served as a holiday food, wrapped in corn husks and served at the table as little bundles filled with delectable flavors. Next time you shuck corn, save the husks and make these tamales for an extra special treat. No need to wait for a holiday! Masa harina is the corn flour used to make tacos and tortillas in Mexico. You should be able to find it in most supermarkets in the aisle selling Latin ingredients.

Serves 4

For the dough:
2 cups masa harina
1 teaspoon baking powder
1 teaspoon salt
6 tablespoons nonfat Greek yogurt
1¾ cups water

For the tamales:
8 large dried cornhusks, soaked for 2 hours in hot water
2 roasted poblano peppers, diced
⅓ cup cilantro leaves

For the garnish:
8 tablespoons crumbled queso fresco or farmer cheese
Salsa or hot sauce (optional)

METHOD To prepare the tamale dough: In a medium mixing bowl, combine the masa harina, baking powder, and salt. Mix well. Add the yogurt and water and stir to form a soft dough.

To prepare the tamales: Divide the dough into 8 to 12 equal portions, depending on how large your corn husks are. Place one in the center of each husk. Press the dough into an even layer in the husk, leaving a 1½-inch border. Add some of the chopped roasted poblano chili pepper and cilantro leaves down the center of the dough. Roll the corn husk into a cylinder and fold the ends over to seal the filling. Repeat with the remaining corn husks, dough, and filling.

Arrange half the tamales in a flat steamer basket and cover with a lid. Add water to a large skillet to a depth of 3 inches; bring to a slow simmer. Place the steamer in the skillet. Steam the tamales for 3 hours, until the husks peel away cleanly. Remove the tamales from the steamer. (You may need to add additional water to the pan to steam for 3 hours.)

ASSEMBLY Just prior to serving, open the corn husks to expose the tamales and sprinkle 1 tablespoon of cheese over the cooked tamale. Serve with salsa or hot sauce, if desired.

Per serving: 283 calories • 5 g fat • 2 g sat fat • 10 mg chol • 775 mg sodium • 50 g carb • 1 g sugar • 6 g fiber • 13 g protein • 216 mg calcium

Baked Polenta with
Tomato Sauce and Ricotta

~~~~~~

I turn to polenta when I am in need of some good, old-fashioned comfort food. I suspect it's because there is not much difference between polenta and the grits I was raised on in North Florida. This simple dish relies once again on my favorite tomato sauce and not much else other than freshly cooked polenta made better than ever with a little added ricotta.

Serves 4

For the tomato sauce:
4 tomatoes
1 medium yellow onion, skin on
1 small bulb garlic
2 tablespoons extra-virgin olive oil
Salt

For the polenta:
1 cup polenta
1 tablespoon extra-virgin olive oil
4 tablespoons chopped fresh basil
½ cup ricotta cheese
Salt and freshly ground black pepper
¼ cup grated Parmesan cheese

For the garnish:
4 tablespoons chopped basil

METHOD To prepare the tomato sauce: Preheat the oven to 425°F.

Place the tomatoes, yellow onion, and garlic in a baking pan. Bake for 45 minutes or until the garlic is soft and the skin is peeling away from the tomatoes. Remove from the oven and cool to room temperature. Remove the skin from the tomatoes and put in a saucepan. Squeeze the garlic out of the bulb and into the tomatoes. Remove the skin from the onion. Coarsely chop the onion and add to the tomatoes. Add the olive oil to the tomatoes and puree with a handheld immersion blender until smooth. You may need to add up to ⅓ cup water if there is not enough liquid. Season with salt.

Warm the tomato sauce just prior to use.

To prepare the polenta: Preheat the oven to 400°F.

In a medium saucepan, bring 3 cups of water to a simmer and stream in the polenta. Whisk together until there are no lumps. Cover with a lid and continue to cook over low heat for 20 minutes, stirring every 3 minutes. Be careful when you go to stir the polenta—it tends to spit out pieces of the cornmeal, which is very hot.

Remove the polenta from the heat and stir in the olive oil and basil. Drop in teaspoon-size pieces of the ricotta cheese. Pour the polenta into an 8-inch square baking pan and spread evenly. Sprinkle with the Parmesan cheese and let sit for 1 hour or until the polenta has firmed up.

Bake the polenta in the oven for 15 minutes or until heated through.

Cut the polenta into 8 equal pieces.

ASSEMBLY Place ½ cup of warm tomato sauce in 4 shallow bowls and top with two pieces of the polenta. Sprinkle with the chopped basil.

Per serving: 375 calories • 18 g fat • 5 g sat fat • 17 mg chol • 491 mg sodium • 43 g carb • 7 g sugar • 6 g fiber • 13 g protein • 251 mg calcium

Slow-Cooked Farro with Asparagus and Pecorino Cheese

~~~~~~

Similar to but not exactly the same as spelt, farro is an ancient grain packed with nutrients, fiber, and a subtle nuttiness that no one can resist. I like to cook it slowly and serve it tossed with springtime's best grassy asparagus stalks cut into bite-size lengths. You might prefer another vegetable, but whatever you choose, it will be filling and satisfying. Shave firm cheese over the top, and dinner is served.

Serves 4

1 cup uncooked farro or wheat berries
12 asparagus stalks, trimmed and blanched
2 tablespoons fresh lemon juice
2 tablespoons extra-virgin olive oil
3 tablespoons chopped fresh basil
Salt and freshly ground black pepper
¼ cup shaved pecorino Romano cheese

METHOD Place the farro in a large saucepan, add 2 cups of water, and cover. Bring to a boil and reduce the heat to a simmer. Cover with the lid slightly ajar and continue to cook for 15 to 20 minutes or until the farro is just al dente. Transfer the farro to a medium mixing bowl and cool to room temperature.

Cut the asparagus into 1-inch-long pieces. Add the asparagus, lemon juice, olive oil, and basil to the mixing bowl with the farro and toss until combined. Season to taste with salt and pepper.

ASSEMBLY Equally divide the farro mixture into four bowls and sprinkle with the shaved pecorino Romano cheese. This can be enjoyed chilled, warm, or even hot.

Per serving: 274 calories • 10 g fat • 3 g sat fat • 8 mg chol • 129 mg sodium • 37 g carb • 2 g sugar • 6 g fiber • 11 g protein • 126 mg calcium

Put the Health Back in Shopping

Trips to the supermarket don't have to be a chore, nor should they be a time for disorganized extravagance. I'm sure you've heard the good advice about never shopping when you're hungry. If you do, you will probably buy more than you need, purchase items not on your list (like ice cream and Oreos), and allow that little voice in your head to convince you it's perfectly okay to try the frozen pizza balls or tub of onion dip.

I don't want to sound too preachy, but because I have spent a good deal of my life in sprawling markets, lively farmer's markets, and specialty gourmet shops, I know a thing or two about shopping. And I'm not talking Rodeo Drive or Michigan Avenue shopping. I'm talking everyday grocery shopping.

If you're organized, if you think about what you and your family like, and if you make an effort to make it through the market without distraction, you will be happier and your family meals will be far more healthful.

Here are my three tips for successful shopping. They will allow you to get in and out of the market efficiently and bring home the best food you can.

First, make a list. If you know what's in your pantry, freezer, and refrigerator, you will be able to keep the list updated.

Second, decide on a few recipes. You know what you like to cook, and once you leaf through this book, you will want to try a few new dishes every week. Make sure you buy what you need for several meals.

Third, know the layout of the market and start with the produce. Markets are arranged so that perishable foods are displayed around the perimeter. This means fruits and vegetables, meat, poultry and fish, and dairy. The inside aisles have boxed and canned foods, frozen foods, and any number of processed and "quick-cooking" offerings.

If you start by buying the whole foods—apples, lettuce, oranges, berries, green beans, bananas, potatoes, and onions—you will be less tempted when you enter the inside aisles. Plan to end your trip with stops at the meat and fish counters and the dairy refrigerators. This way, the most perishable foods will be in the cart for the shortest length of time.

When you buy canned and frozen foods, read the labels. Choose items with small amounts of sodium and sugars. Avoid fruits packed in syrup. Go for low fat and low calories. Understand how the serving sizes are figured.

Most importantly, make an effort to buy food in its most natural state. Whole. Fresh. Ripe. And don't buy more than you and your family can eat within five or six days.

Augment your supermarket purchases with items you buy at the local farmer's market or farm stand, paying attention to when specific fruits and veggies are in season. Not only will the produce taste better, but the price will be right.

You might want to find a specialty market with a good butcher or fish counter so that you can be sure you are buying responsibly raised poultry and meat, and perhaps line-caught fish.

Once you get in the habit of cooking with whole foods, you will enjoy it. Best of all, you will know your family is eating healthfully. ❊

Shirataki Noodles Stir-Fry

Stir-fries are a great way to get your veggies, and when they are augmented with noodles, you have a full meal. Shirataki noodles were a happy discovery. Made from yam flour, they are extremely low in calories and fat, but bulk up the stir-fry just the way I like it. Compare these to a cup of regular spaghetti, which has about 220 calories, and you'll grab the shiratakis, too. Look for plastic pouches of them in stores like Whole Foods and in Asian markets.

Serves 4

For the noodles:
2 tablespoons canola oil
1 tablespoon chopped garlic
1 tablespoon chopped fresh ginger
1 jalapeno pepper, seeded and minced
6 stalks rapini (also called broccoli rabe), coarsely chopped
1 cup shredded carrots
4 cups sliced shiitake mushrooms
½ cup almond milk
1 teaspoon sriracha or another hot sauce
2 tablespoons low-sodium soy sauce
2 8-ounce bags shirataki noodles, drained and rinsed

For the garnish:
½ cup chopped green onions
½ cup chopped peanuts
4 tablespoons cilantro leaves
1 lime, quartered

METHOD In a wok or large sauté pan, warm the oil over medium-high heat. Add the garlic, ginger, and jalapeno pepper to the pan and cook for 1 to 2 minutes or until fragrant. Add the rapini, carrots, and mushrooms and cook for 5 minutes or until the mushrooms are tender. Add the almond milk, hot sauce, soy sauce, and noodles. Cook for 2 minutes or until the noodles are hot. Remove from the heat.

ASSEMBLY Divide the noodles among 4 serving plates and sprinkle with the green onions, peanuts, and cilantro leaves. Squeeze the lime juice over the noodles.

Per serving: 254 calories • 17 g fat • 2 g sat fat • 0 mg chol • 373 mg sodium • 19 g carb • 5 g sugar • 5 g fiber • 10 g protein • 188 mg calcium

Stir-fried dishes are always best when made at the very last moment. They just take minutes to cook and when enjoyed fresh out of the pan the results are always a hit! Buckwheat soba noodles or rice noodles are a great substitution for the shirataki noodles. I like to jazz up this dish with more heat and I am always happy to have my bottle of sriracha sauce nearby.

Potato Tart with Mustard Greens and Lemon Thyme

~~~~~~~~~~~~~~~~~~~~~~~~~~~~~~~~~~

The beautiful kitchen in my Chicago house was designed by Canadian designer Kevin Fitzsimons, who is a devout Buddhist. Kevin and I became friends, and when I mentioned to him that I would love to cook for His Holiness the Dalai Lama, he came through. When the Dalai Lama visited Toronto for an official Canadian visit, Kevin arranged for me to cook a meal for him. I enlisted the help of vegan chef Tal Ronnen and the chef at my Chicago restaurant, Rey Villalobos. Together we came up with a meal that included Canada's best fresh fruits and vegetables as well as a vegan "fried chicken" made from a Gardein product (Gardein makes superior vegetable-based food products). The Dalai Lama loved the meal and personally thanked us. That moment was one of the highlights of my life. When I was booted from *Top Chef Masters* in the Vegan Challenge one season, I was consoled by the memory of the Dalai Lama being so appreciative of my vegan cuisine!

While this tart was not on the menu that evening, I am thrilled to see whole wheat phyllo dough in the markets. It's so much better for you than phyllo made with processed white flour and makes a crispy crust for this lively potato tart. I say "lively" because the flavors of mustard greens, lemon thyme, and goat cheese enliven the potatoes to create a treat worth making.

Serves 6

4 sheets whole wheat phyllo dough
1 large Yukon Gold potato, sliced paper thin
½ cup buttermilk
Salt and freshly ground black pepper
1 tablespoon canola oil
½ cup chopped onion
2 cups chopped mustard greens
2 large eggs
3 large egg whites
½ cup skim milk
2 teaspoons lemon thyme leaves
2 ounces soft goat cheese (about 4 tablespoons)

METHOD Preheat the oven to 375°F.

Line a 10-inch tart pan with the whole wheat phyllo dough. Leave a ½-inch overhang and trim any excess. Place the tart pan on a baking sheet.

In a medium mixing bowl, toss the potato slices with the buttermilk and season with salt and pepper.

In a large sauté pan, heat the canola oil over medium heat and add the onions. Cook the onions for 2 minutes over medium-high heat. Add the mustard greens to the pan and cook for 5 minutes or until they are wilted. Season with salt and pepper.

Shingle half the potato slices on the bottom of the phyllo-lined tart pan. Sprinkle with half of the mustard greens. Repeat the process with the remaining potatoes and mustard greens.

In a medium bowl, whisk the eggs, egg whites, and skim milk for 1 minute or until combined. Add the lemon thyme and season with salt and pepper. Pour the egg mixture over the potatoes. Drop teaspoons of the goat cheese around the tart.

Bake the tart for 45 to 60 minutes or until it is just set and the potatoes are cooked. Remove from the oven and let sit for 15 minutes before cutting.

ASSEMBLY Cut the tart into 6 pieces and place on a serving plate.

Per serving: 272 calories • 10 g fat • 4 g sat fat • 116 mg chol • 260 mg sodium • 32 g carb • 5 g sugar • 3 g fiber • 13 g protein • 148 mg calcium

How Much Fruits and Vegetables?

I don't think most of us need to worry about eating too many vegetables. We might need to put on the brakes if faced with a bushel basket of perfectly ripe, juicy peaches or crispy fall apples, but it's unlikely you'll overdose on fruit either.

There's a greater chance you aren't eating enough vegetables and fruit. Seventy-five percent of Americans don't get the recommended daily amount of either. And too many of us think a baked potato and a glass of lemonade meet the grade.

According to the experts, we should eat *at least* two and a half cups of vegetables and two cups of fruit every day. Some nutritionists think we should eat a whole lot more. The USDA determines that a half cup of either is a serving—with two obvious exceptions: a serving of lettuce is twice that, and a serving of dried fruit is half.

There are lots of ways to work enough vegetables and fruits into your daily diet without walking around with a measuring cup in your pocket. Here are a few:

✦ Cover half your plate with vegetables and fruit at every meal.

✦ Slice up an apple or orange to eat with lunch and dinner.

✦ Cut back on servings of potatoes; eat legumes, whole grains, and sweet potatoes instead. These carbs are digested more slowly, which is a good thing.

✦ Munch on baby carrots, which travel well to work and school.

✦ Keep fruit in a bowl on the counter so you are reminded to eat it.

✦ Take an apple or a couple of clementines to the office for a midafternoon snack.

✦ Make sure to include sliced banana or berries on your morning cereal.

✦ Toss dried cranberries or blueberries in your salads or granola.

✦ Try the various brands of veggie burgers on the market, and eat them several times a month or more.

- ✦ Add grated or sliced apples or pears to turkey burgers and meat loaf.

- ✦ Make green salads with lots of added veggies, such as bell peppers, radishes, sugar snap peas, and onions.

- ✦ Make smoothies with low-fat yogurt and fresh or frozen unsweetened fruit.

- ✦ Load up pizzas with veggie toppings.

- ✦ Always add lettuce and tomatoes to sandwiches—and think about peppers, onions, and crunchy radishes and sprouts, too.

- ✦ Cut up broccoli, cauliflower, carrots, cucumbers, and other veggies to eat with light yogurt-based dips.

- ✦ Make your own salsa or, barring that, buy your favorite brand. Spoon it over burgers, eggs, and chicken breasts, and use it to moisten sandwiches.

- ✦ Grill extra veggies every time you grill and keep them on hand for veggie sandwiches. Some that are especially good are sliced eggplant, summer squash, asparagus, bell peppers, portobello mushrooms, and onions.

- ✦ Roast winter vegetables, which take on an irresistible sweetness in the oven, and eat them with everything for a few days: eggs, chicken breasts, fish, sandwiches— you name it! I especially like to roast onions, turnips, beets, and cauliflower.

- ✦ Keep a supply of canned and frozen fruits and vegetables in the kitchen. Make sure they are not packed in syrup or sauces. Even canned or frozen, they retain much of their nutritional value.

- ✦ Buy bagged greens, precut butternut squash, and other partially prepped ingredients. If doing so persuades you to eat more of these vegetables, I am all for it.

But why? Why make such an effort to eat vegetables and fruits? They protect our hearts, help keep blood pressure within healthful boundaries, protect against a number of cancers, and keep our bodies well regulated.

Need *more* encouragement? They taste good! ❈

Dirty Rice with Mushroom Bolognese

~~~~~~

Dirty rice is a wacky name for a delicious dish. Coming from Cajun country, it refers to rice cooked with chicken livers that darken it so it looks "dirty." No chicken livers in this one, but I make a Bolognese with brown cremini mushrooms that I then spoon over brown rice cooked in the mushroom stock. Very tasty! And the color of the entire dish earns it the name "dirty." We serve this at Art and Soul in D.C., where folks find it soul satisfying!

Serves 4

For the mushroom Bolognese:
12 ounces cremini mushrooms, cleaned (about 3 cups)
½ cup chopped minced carrots
½ cup chopped minced yellow onion
½ cup chopped celery
2 tablespoons extra-virgin olive oil

For the dirty rice:
1 cup short-grain brown rice
6 cups hot mushroom stock or water
¼ cup chopped flat-leaf parsley
¼ cup grated Parmesan cheese
Salt and freshly ground black pepper

For the garnish:
4 teaspoons extra-virgin olive oil
2 tablespoons chopped fresh basil

METHOD To prepare the mushroom Bolognese: Place the mushrooms, carrots, yellow onion, and celery in a food processor fitted with a metal blade. Process until finely chopped.

Warm the olive oil in a large sauté pan over medium heat. Add the mushroom mixture and cook over very low heat for about 60 to 90 minutes or until all the liquid is cooked out of the mushrooms, they turn a nice dark color, and the vegetables are tender.

To prepare the dirty rice: Place the brown rice in a shallow saucepan and add ½ cup of the stock. Cook over low heat while constantly stirring until all the liquid is absorbed into the rice. Continue to add the stock in ½-cup additions, stirring all the while, until the rice is creamy and cooked al dente (about 45 minutes). This cooking method is similar to cooking risotto.

Add the mushroom Bolognese to the rice and cook for 5 minutes over low heat to infuse the flavors. Stir in parsley and Parmesan cheese and season with salt and pepper.

ASSEMBLY Divide the dirty rice among 4 serving plates, drizzle the olive oil around the rice, and sprinkle with the chopped basil.

Per serving: 342 calories • 14 g fat • 3 g sat fat • 4 mg chol • 118 mg sodium • 46 g carb • 3 g sugar • 4 g fiber • 9 g protein • 123 mg calcium

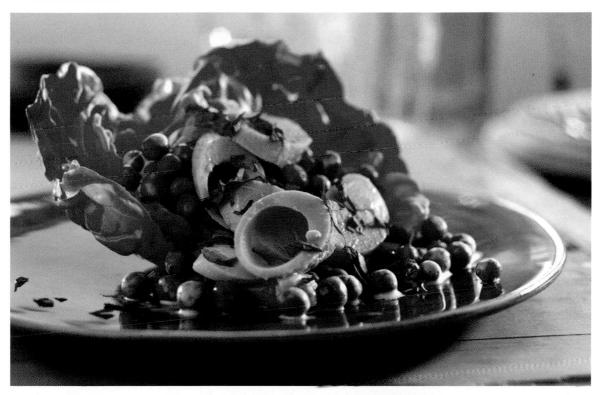

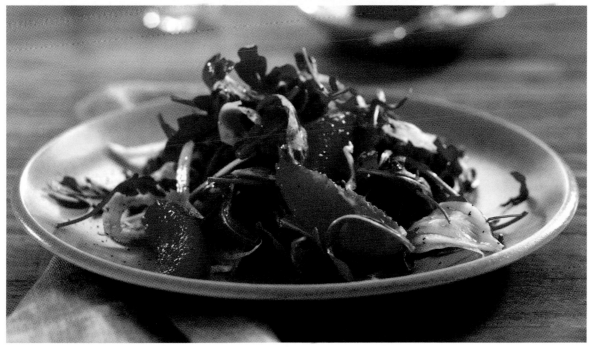

✻ *Top:* CHILLED PEAS WITH HEART OF PALM, BASIL, AND YOGURT (page 70) ✻
✻ *Bottom:* FRESH FENNEL AND ARUGULA WITH MEYER LEMON DRESSING (page 72) ✻

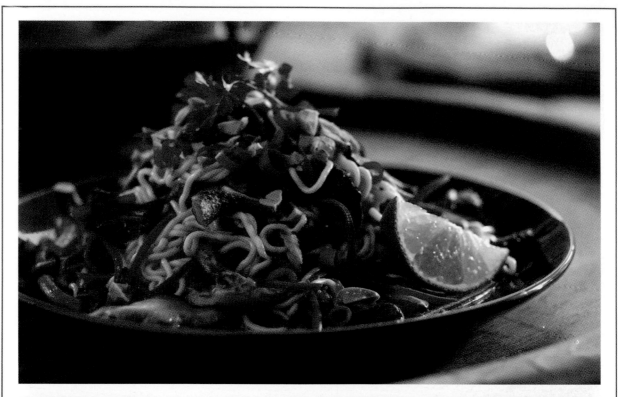

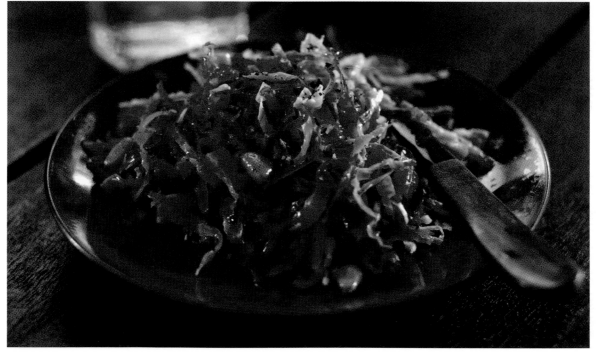

※ *Top:* SHIRATAKI NOODLES STIR-FRY (page 106) ※
※ *Bottom:* SHAVED BRUSSELS SPROUT SALAD WITH PINE NUTS AND LEMON (page 90) ※

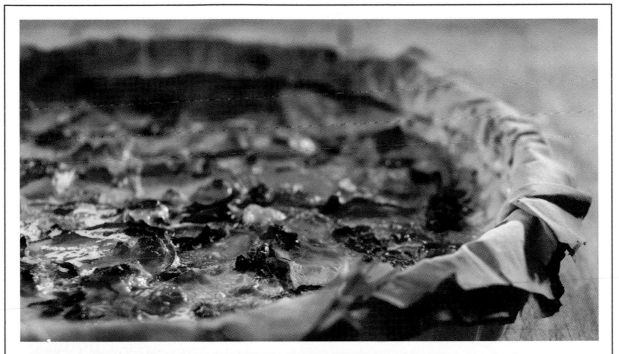

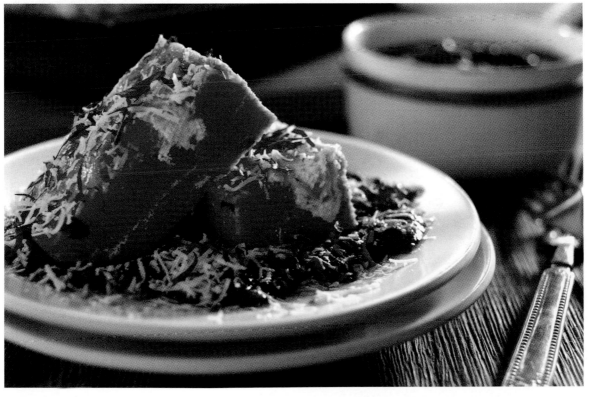

❋ *Top:* POTATO TART WITH MUSTARD GREENS AND LEMON THYME (page 108) ❋
❋ *Bottom:* BAKED POLENTA WITH TOMATO SAUCE AND RICOTTA (page 102) ❋

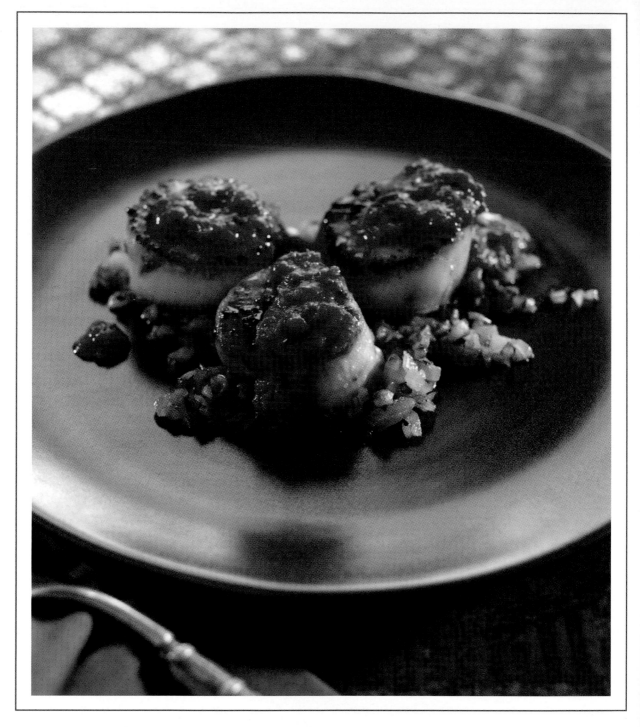

✳ LIME AND MINT SCALLOPS WITH RED ONION (page 118) ✳

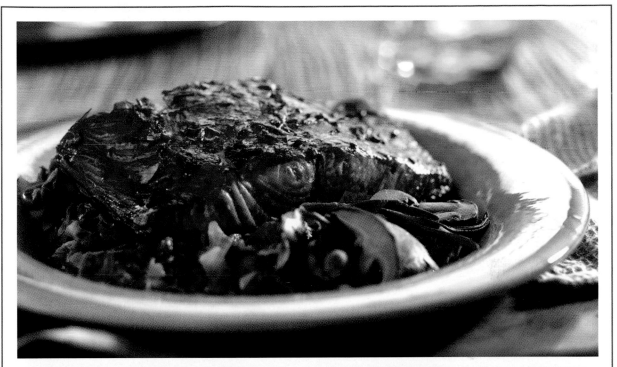

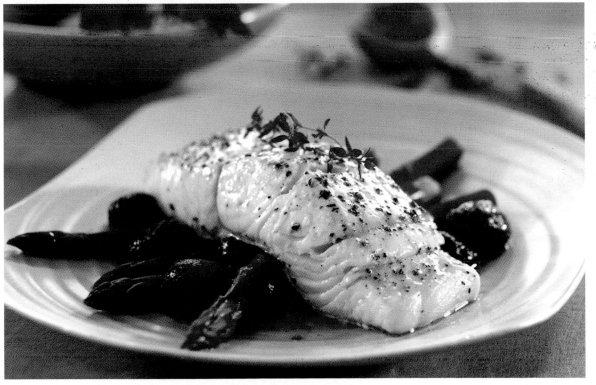

❋ *Top:* BROILED SALMON WITH WILD MUSHROOMS AND LENTILS (page 120) ❋
❋ *Bottom:* HALIBUT WITH ROASTED TOMATOES AND ASPARAGUS (page 124) ❋

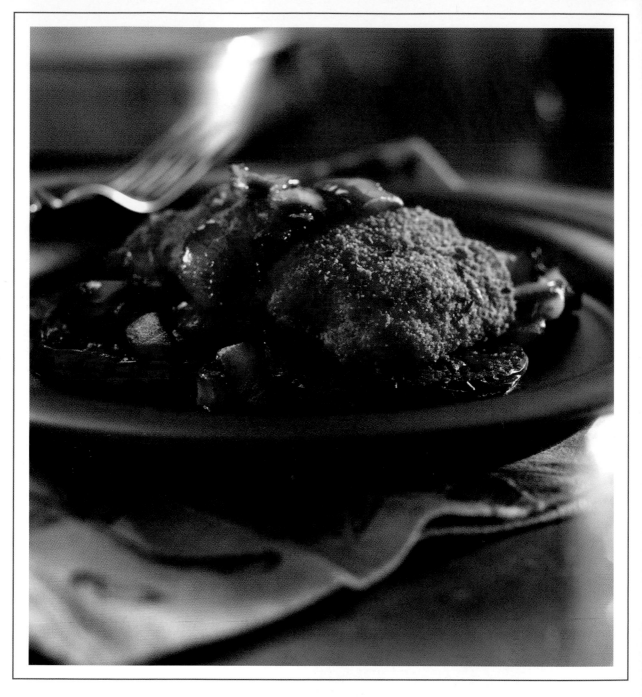

※ CORNMEAL-CRUSTED CATFISH WITH GREEN TOMATOES AND VIDALIA ONIONS (page 126) ※

Fish and Seafood Main Courses

~~~~~~

When I was growing up, fried catfish was as ordinary as fried chicken. We lived in Jasper, a small rural town close to Florida's panhandle that was near both the ocean and the Suwannee River, so seafood, both saltwater and freshwater, was commonplace. A catfish supper at church or a community center was a regular occurrence and one I always enjoyed. When done right, fried catfish is out of this world. These days, I try to stay away from anything fried, even catfish, and don't miss it one bit when I dig into the Cornmeal-Crusted Catfish with Green Tomatoes and Vidalia Onions on page 126.

Finfish and, to a lesser degree, seafood (clams, oysters, mussels, scallops, shrimp, crayfish, crabs, and lobster) are really good for us. They are low in fat and high in protein. The fattier fishes (tuna, salmon, sardines, trout, and cod) are excellent sources of omega-3 fatty acids, which benefit our hearts. Seafood is slightly less beneficial because it can raise cholesterol levels, but shrimp, crabs, and scallops are also good ways to get omega-3s. Risk of exposure to mercury is minimal in most cases, although pregnant women should limit their consumption of fish and seafood and of course talk to their doctors about it. Most nutritionists and scientists feel the overall benefits far outweigh any risks and suggest we eat fish twice a week. I agree!

The trick to getting the most from fish and seafood is to buy it fresh. If you live near the ocean and know a local seafood vendor who buys it "off the boat," lucky you. Even better, if you like to fish you will be richly rewarded. You may like to fish from a boat on the ocean or on one of our Great Lakes, or prefer to wade into a rushing brook and cast for trout. I am not a fisherman, but when friends share their just-caught fish with me, I am blown away by the amazing flavor.

Most of us don't have the luxury of buying fish right off the boat or catching our own and so must depend on fish stores and fish counters in supermarkets. Talk to the guy selling the fish to find out what is freshest that day. And when the fish counter doesn't catch your fancy on any given day, don't shy away from frozen fish. A lot of it is high quality, especially given today's technology, which allows fresh-caught fish to be flash-frozen while the fishing vessel is still at sea. Farmed fish is another option. The people who farm fish have made great strides in recent years, and the risk of pollutants in the waters where the fish is raised has been reduced and the farmers are more careful about what they feed their fish. Plus, we can't continue to deplete our fish stocks in the open sea, so farmed fish (carp, catfish, salmon, and tilapia) and farmed seafood (clams, oysters, scallops, and mussels) are the way of the future. Support fish farmers who are trying to get it right.

*L*ime and Mint Scallops with Red Onion ✳ 118

*B*roiled Salmon with Wild Mushrooms and Lentils ✳ 120

*P*resident Barack Obama's Favorite Glazed Salmon ✳ 122

*H*alibut with Roasted Tomatoes and Asparagus ✳ 124

*C*ornmeal-Crusted Catfish with Green Tomatoes and Vidalia Onions ✳ 126

*T*rout with Roasted Red Beets, Radishes, and Dill Dressing ✳ 128

*S*wordfish with Capers, Olives, Tomato Sauce, and Whole Wheat Penne ✳ 130

*F*ish Tacos with Chayote Slaw and Chipotle Aioli ✳ 132

*B*roiled Sea Bass with Ginger, Garlic, and Carrots ✳ 134

*R*oasted Tilapia with Lemon and Cilantro ✳ 136

*S*teel-Cut Oatmeal Risotto with Shrimp and Sweet Peas ✳ 138

*S*hrimp and Hominy ✳ 140

*S*teamed Mussels with Ginger and Thai Red Chilies ✳ 142

Lime and Mint Scallops with Red Onion

~~~~~~

Scallops and mint taste lovely together, one so mild and the other delightfully piquant, but beyond that obvious attraction, what I love about this dish is its versatility. I usually serve it warm directly after cooking, but through trial and error I discovered it tastes just as spectacular if served at room temp or even chilled. So, make this often and serve it when it fits into your schedule.

Serves 4

For the mint sauce:
1 cup shucked peas
½ cup fresh mint leaves
2 tablespoons fresh lime juice
Salt and freshly ground black pepper

For the scallops:
12 large sea scallops
Salt and freshly ground black pepper
1 to 2 tablespoons extra-virgin olive oil
1 large red onion, minced

METHOD **To prepare the mint sauce:** Blanch the peas in a pot of boiling salted water for 3 minutes. Drain immediately and shock in a bowl of ice water. Drain and transfer the peas to a food processor fitted with a metal blade. Add the mint leaves and lime juice and pulse a few times or until the mixture is somewhat chunky. Season with salt and pepper. Keep at room temperature or refrigerate until ready to use.

To prepare the scallops: Season the scallops with salt and pepper. Place 1 tablespoon olive oil in a preheated large nonstick sauté pan. Add the scallops to the pan (if they don't all fit, cook them in 2 or 3 batches). Cook the scallops for 2 to 3 minutes on each side or until they have a nice sear and are golden brown. Remove the scallops from the pan and immediately add the onion to the same pan. If the pan is dry, add the remaining tablespoon of olive oil. Cook the onions for 5 to 7 minutes or until they begin to caramelize.

ASSEMBLY In the center of each plate, spoon some of the onion mixture and top with three scallops. Spoon a tablespoon of the mint sauce over each scallop and enjoy.

Per serving: 145 calories • 7 g fat • 1 g sat fat • 15 mg chol • 75 mg sodium • 10 g carb • 2 g sugar • 2 g fiber • 10 g protein • 28 mg calcium

Spring and summer peas are a special treat. I have always enjoyed snacking on them picked fresh from the field. When the peas get larger in size they tend to develop more starch and those larger peas are best cooked before enjoying. Peas and mint sing together and a few drops of lime or lemon juice brightens the flavors of the peas and mint.

Broiled Salmon with Wild Mushrooms and Lentils

Salmon is the most perfect fish swimming in the sea—and my favorite. It's delish, it's satisfying, and it's packed with heart-healthy omega-3 fatty acids and vitamin D. According to some studies, it also protects the joints, makes the insulin your body naturally secretes highly effective, and aids digestion. Wow! Who wouldn't eat salmon? A lot of the available salmon is farmed, and over the years farmed fish got a bad name. The industry listened and practices have improved, and since many of our oceans are overfished, fish farming is the future. When you see wild-caught salmon in the markets, buy it, but at other times, buy it from a reputable vendor who in turn buys from reputable fish farms. Whatever you do, don't skip eating salmon!

Serves 4

For the lentils:
2 teaspoons extra-virgin olive oil
½ cup chopped yellow onion
2 cups low-sodium chicken stock or water
1 cup French green lentils
1½ ounces prosciutto, julienned
2 tablespoons chopped flat-leaf parsley
Salt and freshly ground black pepper

For the mushrooms:
4 cups wild mushrooms (such as creminis, oysters, or chanterelles)
1 sprig rosemary
2 cloves garlic
Salt and freshly ground black pepper

For the salmon:
4 6-ounce pieces of salmon, skin and bones removed
4 teaspoons low-sodium soy sauce
½ cup minced red onion
1 lemon, quartered

For the garnish:
1 tablespoon chopped flat-leaf parsley

METHOD **To prepare the lentils:** Place the olive oil in a medium sauce-pan and warm over medium heat. Add the onion to the pan and cook over medium-high heat for 3 to 4 minutes or until translucent. Add the chicken stock and the lentils to the pan, and bring to a slow simmer. Continue to simmer for 20 to 40 minutes (older lentils take longer to cook than younger lentils), or until the lentils are tender. Remove from the heat and fold in the prosciutto and chopped parsley. Season with salt and pepper.

To prepare the mushrooms: Preheat the oven to 350°F.

Wash the mushrooms under cold water and trim and discard the ends of the stems. Cut the mushrooms in half and place in a small baking dish with the rosemary and garlic. Add ¼ cup water. Cover with aluminum foil and bake in the oven for 30 to 45 minutes or until just cooked. Remove the mushrooms from the oven and season with salt and pepper.

To prepare the salmon: Preheat the broiler.

Rub the salmon with the soy sauce and top with an even coating of the red onion. Place on a nonstick broiling pan or baking dish with low sides. Broil the salmon for 10 minutes or until cooked medium.

Remove the salmon from the oven and squeeze the lemon over it.

ASSEMBLY In the center of each plate, spoon some of the cooked lentils and mushrooms. Top with a piece of the salmon and sprinkle with the parsley.

Per serving: 529 calories • 18 g fat • 3 g sat fat • 116 mg chol • 596 mg sodium • 37 g carb • 4 g sugar • 8 g fiber • 57 g protein • 77 mg calcium

President Barack Obama's
Favorite Glazed Salmon

~~~~~~~~~~~~~~~~~~~~~~~~~~~~~~~~~~~~~

President Obama and First Lady Michelle Obama are neighbors of mine in Chicago, and I am proud to say that since Oprah introduced us a while ago I have cooked more than one family meal for them. The President particularly likes this teriyaki-style glaze, which makes sense since he grew up in Hawaii, where Asian-inspired foods are prevalent. My longtime friend Hawaiian chef Alan Wong and I worked on this recipe together, which pleases folks on both sides of the aisle. When you make the glaze with fresh ginger and top-rate Dijon mustard, it practically sings out loud. The sesame seeds are an inspired final touch. Putting a sweet glaze on fish is a good way to get everyone, even kids, to dig in!

Serves 8

For the glaze:
1 tablespoon brown sugar
2 teaspoons unsalted butter
1 teaspoon honey
1 tablespoon extra-virgin olive oil
1 tablespoon Dijon mustard
1 tablespoon reduced-sodium soy sauce
1 tablespoon grated fresh ginger
1 teaspoon sesame seeds

For the salmon:
1 salmon fillet (2½ pounds), skin on, pin bones removed
Salt and freshly ground black pepper

METHOD **To prepare the glaze:** In a small saucepan over medium heat, heat the brown sugar, butter, and honey, stirring, until melted. Remove from the heat and whisk in the oil, mustard, soy sauce, ginger, and sesame seeds. Cool for 5 minutes.

To prepare the salmon: Preheat the oven to 350°F.
Place the salmon in a large foil-lined baking pan and season with

salt and pepper. Spoon the glaze over the salmon. Bake uncovered for 20 to 25 minutes or until the fish flakes easily with a fork.

ASSEMBLY Place the salmon on a serving platter and serve hot or at room temperature.

Per serving: 267 calories • 13 g fat • 2 g sat fat • 92 mg chol • 183 mg sodium • 3 g carb • 2 g sugar • 0 g fiber • 32 g protein • 21 mg calcium

---

Oftentimes when I entertain I enjoy setting up a beautiful buffet on my kitchen island or outdoor patio. If you are having a large group of guests it is nice to display a whole side of salmon. A perfectly glazed side of salmon is a showstopper and it can be enjoyed hot right out of the oven or at room temperature. Leftover pieces can be refrigerated and topped on a bed of lettuces for your lunch the next day.

Halibut with Roasted Tomatoes and Asparagus

Halibut can be pulled from the Atlantic or Pacific Ocean. Wherever it's pulled from the deep, it's a magnificent fish. I am drawn to its mild but distinct flavor, and like most white-fleshed fish, it is low in saturated fat and high in protein. At my D.C. restaurant, Art and Soul, the cherry tomatoes we roast are very similar to these. They taste great with the halibut!

Serves 4

For the tomatoes:
24 cherry tomatoes
6 cloves garlic, smashed
2 tablespoons fresh lemon juice
2 tablespoons extra-virgin olive oil
2 sprigs thyme

For the halibut:
4 6-ounce pieces of halibut, skin and bones removed
4 teaspoons extra-virgin olive oil
Salt and freshly ground black pepper

For the asparagus:
16 stalks asparagus, ends trimmed

For the garnish:
4 teaspoons chopped chives or basil
1 lemon, quartered

METHOD **To prepare the tomatoes:** Preheat the oven to 250°F.

Score the tops of the tomatoes with a knife. Place the tomatoes, garlic cloves, lemon juice, olive oil, and thyme in a small ovenproof pan (you do not want lots of extra room in the pan). Cover the pan with aluminum foil. Slowly roast the tomatoes in the oven for 2 hours or until the skins are pulling away. Discard the thyme sprigs and tomato skins.

To prepare the halibut: Preheat the oven to 425°F.

Place the halibut on a nonstick baking sheet. Rub the halibut with the olive oil and season with salt and pepper. Bake for 20 minutes or until cooked through.

To prepare the asparagus: Bring a pot of salted water to a boil and cook the asparagus for 3 to 4 minutes or until al dente. Remove the asparagus from the pot and use immediately.

ASSEMBLY Place 4 asparagus stalks on each plate and spoon 6 of the roasted tomatoes over the asparagus. Place a piece of the halibut in the center of each serving. Sprinkle with the chopped chives or basil and squeeze the lemon juice over the halibut.

Per serving: 340 calories • 16 g fat • 2 g sat fat • 54 mg chol • 99 mg sodium • 13 g carb • 5 g sugar • 5 g fiber • 39 g protein • 136 mg calcium

Cornmeal-Crusted Catfish with
Green Tomatoes and Vidalia Onions

~~~~~~

This recipe comes right out of my southern childhood, although back then we'd fry the catfish, while here I bake it. Across the South we eat green tomatoes to make the most of the abundant tomato crop, and mild Vidalia onions are grown in and around Vidalia, Georgia. Southern cooking all the way, baby!

Serves 4

For the catfish:
4 8-ounce catfish fillets, skin and bones removed
1½ cups buttermilk
1 cup cornmeal
2 tablespoons chopped flat-leaf parsley
1 tablespoon smoked paprika
Salt

For the green tomatoes:
2 medium green tomatoes
1 tablespoon extra-virgin olive oil
1 tablespoon balsamic vinegar
Salt and freshly ground black pepper

For the sweet onions:
1 large Vidalia onion
1 tablespoon extra-virgin olive oil
1 teaspoon balsamic vinegar
Salt and freshly ground black pepper
2 tablespoons chopped chives

For the garnish:
1 lemon, quartered (optional)

METHOD To prepare the catfish: Place the catfish fillets in a bowl and cover with the buttermilk. Refrigerate for 6 hours.

Preheat the oven to 425°F. Line a baking sheet with parchment paper.

Place the cornmeal in a medium mixing bowl and stir in the parsley, smoked paprika, and ¼ teaspoon salt. Remove the catfish from the buttermilk and put it in the bowl. Turn the catfish so it is well coated on all sides. Place the cornmeal-crusted catfish on the prepared sheet and bake in the oven for 12 minutes, or until the fish feels firm to the touch and is cooked all the way through.

To prepare the tomatoes and onions: Preheat the broiler.

Slice the tomatoes into ½-inch-thick slices. Place in a mixing bowl with the olive oil and vinegar. Lay the slices on a broiling pan and broil for 3 to 5 minutes or until the tomatoes begin to caramelize. Remove from the broiler and season to taste with salt and pepper.

Slice the Vidalia onion into ½-inch-thick rings. Lay flat on a non-stick baking sheet and drizzle with the olive oil and balsamic vinegar. Season with salt and freshly ground black pepper. Place under the broiler and cook for 5 to 6 minutes or until the onions are slightly charred. Remove from the broiler and cool slightly. Coarsely chop the onions and toss with the juices that remain on the baking sheet or the cutting board. Fold in the chives.

ASSEMBLY Place 2 to 3 tomato slices on each plate and place the cooked catfish over the tomatoes. Spoon the chopped onion mixture over the catfish.

Squeeze additional lemon juice over the catfish if desired.

Per serving: 511 calories • 15 g fat • 3 g sat fat • 135 mg chol • 213 mg sodium • 48 g carb • 12 g sugar • 3 g fiber • 45 g protein • 171 mg calcium

Trout with Roasted Red Beets, Radishes, and Dill Dressing

~~~~~~

If you've ever fished in one of America's thousands of streams and small rivers and hooked a trout, you know how delicious they are just hours out of the water. You don't have to catch your own fish to enjoy this recipe, which is one we serve often at Art and Soul. The gentle trout tastes wonderful with the sweet, roasted beets and light dill dressing.

Serves 4

For the beets:
16 baby beets
2 tablespoons red wine vinegar
2 teaspoons honey

For the dill dressing:
6 tablespoons extra-virgin olive oil
¼ cup chopped fresh dill
1 tablespoon minced shallot
1 tablespoon fresh lemon juice
1 tablespoon champagne vinegar
Salt and freshly ground pepper

For the trout:
4 6-ounce pieces of trout, skin on, bones removed
Salt and freshly ground black pepper
1 tablespoon extra-virgin olive oil

For the garnish:
4 radishes, thinly sliced

METHOD **To prepare the beets:** Preheat the oven to 425°F.

Trim the stems from the beets, but leave the skin intact. Wrap the beets in aluminum foil and place on a baking sheet. Bake the beets for 30 minutes or until tender. Remove from the oven and cool to room temperature. Once the beets are cooked, the skins will easily come off when rubbed with a paper towel. Cut the beets in half and place in a small mixing bowl. Toss with the vinegar and honey.

To prepare the dressing: Place the olive oil, dill, shallot, lemon juice, and vinegar in a mason jar fitted with a lid. Secure the lid and shake until combined. Season with salt and pepper.

To prepare the trout: Season the trout with salt and pepper. Place the olive oil in a preheated large nonstick sauté pan over medium-high heat. Add the trout to the pan and cook for 4 minutes on each side or until golden brown and cooked through. Remove the trout from the pan and immediately add the beets and the juices from the bowl. Toss the beets in the pan and cook for 2 minutes over medium heat or until warm.

ASSEMBLY Place a piece of the trout on each plate. Spoon some of the beets over the trout and sprinkle the radishes over the beets. Drizzle the dressing over the beets and radishes.

Per serving: 599 calories • 36 g fat • 6 g sat fat • 97 mg chol • 315 mg sodium • 32 g carb • 23 g sugar • 8 g fiber • 40 g protein • 122 mg calcium

Swordfish with Capers, Olives, Tomato Sauce, and Whole Wheat Penne

Years ago when Oprah opened the Oprah Winfrey Leadership Academy for Girls in Henley-on-Klip, Meyerton, South Africa, people came from all over the world to celebrate her amazing accomplishment. Sidney Poitier, an actor I had long admired, was one of the guests. When I saw him standing alone at the party, I asked if I could cook anything for him. "I eat very clean, Art," he said. I ran off to the giant kitchen in the Palace Hotel in Sun City, South Africa, and whipped up grilled local fish, green vegetables, and some grains. The actor was grateful. Another lesson I learned from Oprah: take care of people and you will be rewarded.

This fish dish is a good way to take care of your family. Pasta and red sauce are always welcome on the dinner table, and this one, topped as it is with rich, flavorful swordfish, is a winner. Swordfish, like salmon, is considered a terrific source of omega-3s and other nutrients. Rather than relying on big swordfish steaks, this recipe uses bite-size pieces because even relatively small amounts provide great taste and great nutrition.

Serves 4

For the tomato sauce:
4 tomatoes
1 medium yellow onion, skin on
1 small bulb garlic
2 tablespoons extra-virgin olive oil
Salt

For the swordfish:
12 ounces swordfish, cut into bite-size pieces
Salt and freshly ground black pepper
1 tablespoon extra-virgin olive oil
2 tablespoons capers, rinsed and chopped
12 kalamata olives, pitted and chopped

For the pasta:
12 ounces whole wheat penne pasta, cooked and kept hot

For the garnish:
8 fresh basil leaves, chopped

METHOD **To prepare the tomato sauce:** Preheat the oven to 425°F.

Place the tomatoes, yellow onion, and garlic in a baking pan. Bake for 45 minutes or until the garlic is soft and the skin is peeling away from the tomatoes. Remove from the oven and cool to room temperature. Remove the skin from the tomatoes and put in a saucepan. Squeeze the garlic out of the bulb onto the tomatoes. Remove the skin from the onion. Coarsely chop the onion and add to the tomatoes. Add the olive oil to the tomatoes and puree with a handheld immersion blender until smooth. You many need to add up to ⅓ cup water if there is not enough liquid. Season with salt.

Warm the tomato sauce just prior to use.

To prepare the swordfish: Season the swordfish with salt and pepper. Place the olive oil in a preheated sauté pan and add the swordfish pieces. Cook the swordfish over medium-high heat for 3 minutes or until cooked. Add the capers and olives to the pan and mix until combined.

ASSEMBLY Divide the cooked pasta among 4 serving bowls. Spoon the tomato sauce over the pasta and top with the swordfish mixture. Sprinkle the basil over the bowl.

Per serving: 582 calories • 19 g fat • 3 g sat fat • 31 mg chol • 406 mg sodium • 75 g carb • 8 g sugar • 10 g fiber • 29 g protein • 74 mg calcium

Fish Tacos with Chayote Slaw and Chipotle Aioli

~~~~~~

Even people who claim they don't like fish, like fish tacos. This is especially true of kids. A lot of parents I know report that their offspring, who turn up their noses at "regular" fish, gobble up fish tacos. I call this a "fish taco" and it can be made with just about any fish. We serve these at LYFE Kitchen where we make them with lovely-tasting mahi mahi. Mahi mahi is the fish's Hawaiian name; in other parts of the country, it is sometimes referred to as dophinfish. Don't worry! No relation to the mammal called a dolphin. But because so many people are confused by the name, the fish, which swims in semitropical and tropical waters, is best known as mahi mahi. And by the way, chayote is a kind of squash grown in warm regions, including Mexico. It is used regularly in Cajun cooking, where it's called mirliton.

Serves 4

For the slaw:
½ cup shredded chayote
1 cup shredded red cabbage
½ cup shredded carrot
½ cup thinly sliced red onion
3 tablespoons fresh lime juice
1 tablespoon extra-virgin olive oil
1 tablespoon agave syrup or stevia
2 teaspoons cider vinegar
¼ teaspoon celery seed
½ teaspoon ground chipotle powder

For the aioli:
½ cup nonfat Greek yogurt
1 teaspoon ground chipotle powder
1 tablespoon fresh lime juice

For the fish:
8 2-ounce pieces of mahi mahi, skin and bones removed
Salt and freshly ground black pepper

For the garnish:
8 6-inch corn tortillas
1 avocado, peeled, seeded, and cut into 16 slices
4 tablespoons cilantro leaves
1 lime, cut into 8 wedges

METHOD **To prepare the slaw:** In a large mixing bowl, combine the chayote, cabbage, carrot, onion, lime juice, olive oil, agave syrup or stevia, vinegar, celery seed, and chipotle powder. Toss together until fully incorporated. Let the flavors marinate for at least 1 hour before serving.

To prepare the aioli: In a small mixing bowl, combine the yogurt, chipotle powder, and lime juice. Refrigerate until ready to use.

To prepare the fish: Preheat the oven to 450°F.

Place the fish on a nonstick baking sheet and season with salt and pepper. Bake in the oven for 5 to 7 minutes or until the fish is just cooked.

ASSEMBLY Place two corn tortillas on each plate. Arrange some of the fish, aioli, and slaw in each tortilla. Top with the avocado slices and cilantro leaves. Garnish with the lime wedges.

Per serving: 389 calories • 12 g fat • 2 g sat fat • 83 mg chol • 209 mg sodium • 45 g carb • 8 g sugar • 7 g fiber • 27 g protein • 73 mg calcium

Broiled Sea Bass with Ginger, Garlic, and Carrots

~~~~~~

I will never forget the night I was cooking dinner for Oprah and her friend Quincy Jones. Turns out, Dr. Dean Ornish was a last-minute guest, and I immediately went into panic mode. Would this great doctor, who believes your diet can change your health, like what I cooked? Because I knew he ate it, I added fish to the menu, which previously had included only chicken. I also drew on Oprah's advice: always offer your guests comfort. The meal was a great success. Although I didn't serve sea bass that night, I might as well have; it's sort of like chicken because it goes with just about everything. In this recipe, I broil the fish, which is a quick and easy way to prepare it without much added fat. The lightly cooked carrots are the perfect garnish for the ginger-tinged fish.

Serves 4

For the carrots:
1 tablespoon extra-virgin olive oil
12 baby carrots, peeled
2 teaspoons honey
Salt and freshly ground black pepper
1 tablespoon chopped flat-leaf parsley

For the sea bass:
4 6-ounce pieces sea bass, skin and bones removed
Salt
¼ cup minced red onion
1 tablespoon minced ginger
1 tablespoon minced garlic
1 tablespoon extra-virgin olive oil
2 teaspoons balsamic vinegar

METHOD To prepare the carrots: Place the olive oil in a preheated large nonstick sauté pan. Add the carrots and cook over medium-high heat for 5 to 7 minutes or until the carrots are tender. Add the honey to the pan and continue to cook for 1 minute. Season with salt and pepper, then add the parsley. Mix until combined.

~~~~~~

To prepare the sea bass: Preheat the broiler.

Season the sea bass with salt and place on a nonstick baking sheet. In a small mixing bowl, combine the onion, ginger, garlic, oil, and vinegar. Spoon the mixture over the top of the sea bass and gently pat it to secure it on the fish. Broil the fish for 7 to 10 minutes or until it is just cooked.

ASSEMBLY Place 3 carrots on each plate and top with a piece of sea bass.

Per serving: 265 calories • 11 g fat • 2 g sat fat • 74 mg chol • 147 mg sodium • 8 g carb • 5 g sugar • 1 g fiber • 33 g protein • 36 mg calcium

Roasted Tilapia with Lemon and Cilantro

What I really love about this recipe is the softened lemon slices that cook along with the fish, lending it a little zing. The Asian-inspired flavors I pair with the tilapia don't overpower the mild fish, but rather accentuate it. This freshwater fish may have originated in North Africa but is now found everywhere, and widely throughout Asia. I suggest buying tilapia from fish farms and managed systems here in the United States. Once you introduce your family to the popular fish, they will welcome it on the table. Its flavor is gentle with just a little sweetness. Perfect!

Serves 4

For the tilapia:
3 lemons, thinly sliced
1½ cups chicken stock
4 6-ounce pieces tilapia, skin and bones removed
Salt
2 jalapeno peppers, minced
2 garlic cloves, minced
2 tablespoons low-sodium soy sauce
1 tablespoon minced ginger
1 tablespoon curry powder
1 tablespoon sesame oil

For the garnish:
¼ cup chopped cilantro
2 green onions, trimmed and chopped

METHOD Preheat the oven to 400°F.

In a large baking dish, lay the lemon slices flat and cover with the chicken stock. Season the tilapia pieces with salt and lay on top of the lemon slices. In a small mixing bowl, combine the jalapeno peppers, garlic, soy sauce, ginger, curry powder, and sesame oil. Spread the mixture over the tilapia. Bake the tilapia for 10 to 15 minutes or until fully cooked.

ASSEMBLY Place a piece of the tilapia on each plate and drizzle the cooking juices over the fish. Sprinkle with the cilantro and green onions, and garnish with the roasted lemon pieces, if desired.

Per serving: 262 calories • 11 g fat • 2 g sat fat • 85 mg chol • 709 mg sodium • 12 g carb • 1 g sugar • 5 g fiber • 36 g protein • 84 mg calcium

Growing up, baked or fried catfish was a regular dish on our family dinner table. Catfish, trout, or even salmon can be used in place of the tilapia in this recipe. It is important to regularly work fish into your diet, and if you bake, grill, or broil it the results will be flavorful as well as healthful.

Don't be afraid to embrace spices in your cooking. The curry, lemon, and cilantro sing together as they bake in the oven with the tilapia and the aromas fill your kitchen, making it inviting for your guests.

Steel-Cut Oatmeal Risotto with Shrimp and Sweet Peas

~~~~~~

What? Savory *oatmeal* risotto? No misprint! It's absolutely delicious and introduces highly nutritious steel-cut oatmeal to the dinner hour. I came up with this for LYFE Kitchen in Northern California, where it's been a big hit. The sautéed shrimp crown the risotto with sweet succulence. And if you have leftover risotto, try it topped with a poached egg for breakfast, brunch, lunch, or supper! Any more questions?

Serves 4

For the oatmeal:
1 tablespoon extra-virgin olive oil
½ cup minced yellow onion
3 cloves garlic, minced
1 cup raw steel-cut oats
3 to 3½ cups hot chicken stock or water
1 cup peas, shucked and blanched
¼ cup grated Parmesan cheese
¼ cup chopped chives
Salt and freshly ground black pepper

For the shrimp:
1 tablespoon extra-virgin olive oil
12 medium shrimp, peeled and deveined
1 tablespoon chopped fresh oregano
1 tablespoon fresh lemon juice

METHOD To prepare the oatmeal: Heat the oil in a large sauté pan. Add the onion and garlic, and cook for 2 minutes or until the onion and garlic are fragrant. Add the oats and cook for 1 minute. Slowly add the hot stock in ¾-cup increments, stirring the oats with a wooden spoon. Continue adding the stock in small amounts until the oats are creamy and cooked al dente. Fold in the peas, Parmesan cheese, and chives. Season with salt and pepper.

To prepare the shrimp: Warm the oil in a preheated large sauté pan. Add the shrimp and cook for 2 minutes on each side or until the shrimp are pink and cooked through. Remove from the heat and toss with the oregano and lemon juice.

ASSEMBLY Divide the oatmeal risotto among 4 bowls and top each with 3 shrimp.

Per serving: 229 calories • 11 g fat • 2 g sat fat • 32 mg chol • 918 mg sodium • 22 g carb • 2 g sugar • 4 g fiber • 11 g protein • 81 mg calcium

Shrimp and Hominy

I'm a son of the South, and while I realize a lot of the food I grew up with is not very healthful, to say the least, I can't stay away from it completely. I developed this recipe for my Atlanta restaurant, Southern Art, taking full advantage of the region's familiarity with hominy, butter beans, and the reality that everything cooked with a little pork tastes "better"! If you don't mind adding some calories, try this over brown rice or grits.

Serves 4

8 ounces dried hominy, soaked overnight in water
¼ cup minced bacon (3 strips)
12 large shrimp, peeled and deveined
1 cup diced tomato
1 cup butter beans (also called lima beans)
4 cloves garlic, chopped
2 cups low-sodium chicken stock
½ cup chopped green onions
1 tablespoon extra-virgin olive oil
Salt and freshly ground black pepper
Hot sauce (optional)

METHOD Drain the hominy, place it in a saucepan, and cover with enough water to reach a depth of 4 inches over the hominy. Bring to a simmer over low heat, season with salt, and cook for 3 to 3½ hours, stirring occasionally, or until the hominy begins to pop open and is tender. You may need to add more water during cooking. Drain the hominy.

In a large sauté pan, cook the bacon over medium-low heat until the fat is rendered. Add the shrimp and cook for 2 minutes. Add the tomato, butter beans, hominy, and garlic. Continue to cook for 2 minutes or until fragrant. Add the chicken stock and allow to simmer for 2 to 4 minutes or until the shrimp are cooked. Add the green onions and olive oil and season with salt and pepper.

ASSEMBLY Divide the shrimp and hominy mixture among 4 bowls and spoon the remaining liquid from the pan into the bowls. Garnish with hot sauce, if desired.

Per serving: 348 calories • 8 g fat • 2 g sat fat • 39 mg chol • 754 mg sodium • 57 g carb • 3 g sugar • 5 g fiber • 14 g protein • 29 mg calcium

---

Hominy! I simply adore and often crave it. Canned hominy can't compare to taking the time to cook dried, uncooked hominy. The textures are incomparable. Hominy often makes me crave pozole, a Mexican stew of hominy, pork, and chicken. But hominy can be coarsely ground to make hominy grits, which are always welcomed in my kitchen!

Steamed Mussels with Ginger and Thai Red Chilies

~~~~~~

All shellfish are great when you're trying to watch your weight because they are extremely low in fat and mussels are one of the best. Granted, the little nugget inside the shiny black shell is no more than a bite, but it's a tasty one, especially when steamed in a fragrant broth.

Serves 4

3 pounds fresh mussels
2 tablespoons extra-virgin olive oil
2 garlic cloves, peeled and thinly sliced
2 shallots, minced
1 tablespoon minced ginger
2 Thai red chilies, thinly sliced
1 cup dry white wine
2 sprigs thyme
Juice of 1 lemon
2 tomatoes, cut into large dice
¼ cup chopped flat-leaf parsley
¼ cup chopped chives

METHOD Rinse mussels under cold running water while scrubbing with a vegetable brush. Pull out the brown beards that stick out of the shell, if necessary. Discard any mussels with cracked or broken shells.

Heat the oil in a large stockpot and warm over medium-high heat. Add the garlic, shallots, ginger, and chilies. Cook for 2 minutes or until fragrant. Add the mussels, wine, thyme, lemon juice, and ½ cup water. Cover the pot and steam over medium-high heat for 5 minutes, until the mussels open. Toss in the tomato, parsley, and chives. Cover the pot and steam for another minute to soften and infuse the flavors.

ASSEMBLY Divide the mussels and broth among 4 serving bowls.

Per serving: 267 calories • 10 g fat • 2 g sat fat • 39 mg chol • 405 mg sodium • 15 g carb • 4 g sugar • 1 g fiber • 18 g protein • 63 mg calcium

Lose the Fat, Keep the Funny

Everyone knows the stereotype of the jolly fat man. Even Santa had "a little round belly, / That shook when he laughed, like a bowl full of jelly!" Kindly, avuncular fat guys are meant to be comforting, but of course not all fat people are kindly or jolly. Many are sad on the inside. I know I was.

When I first started appearing with Oprah on her television show, I hid behind the persona of a funny guy who may have been overweight but at least was "real," and, hey! he liked food. I carried this with me on to *Iron Chef America* and *Top Chef*. This was who I was. Sure, a good guy, but also someone who apparently didn't mind being chunky and who was always ready with a self-deprecating quip about the amount of food he could pack away.

Who could blame me? Even today I don't blame that guy who was me. It feels a lot better to laugh than to cry, right? But as I explore in the introduction to this book, early on I fell into the all-too-familiar trap of eating to feel better, to ease some very real psychic pain. I grew up in a small southern town where being "different" was misunderstood. I was a confused child who grew into a gay man who had a hard time accepting the lifestyle that would accept me. I was bullied as a kid, and when I decided to pursue the life of a cook, my family had a hard time understanding it. It has all worked out now, but for years I suffered in silence. And stuffed my face.

When I lost the weight, I felt as though an oversized overcoat had been removed. Sure, I felt healthy and strong without the extra layers, but I also felt exposed. And oh, how I worried that the funny was gone! In its place was a serious, sensitive man with a host of vulnerabilities as rawly exposed as a Chicagoan is exposed to the winter winds howling off Lake Michigan.

Truth be told, I have not lost my sense of humor and have gained a more rounded, secure, and wise outlook on life and its many lessons. On the one hand, what fun would it be if I couldn't laugh at life or joke with friends and television hosts alike? On the other hand, my heart goes out to those obese folks who are trying to eat away their pain. I hear you! I know you! You are the reason I wrote this book. ❈

Meat and Poultry Main Courses

A good diet, like a good life, is rich in diversity. If you're an omnivore, meat and poultry offer a lot of choices. As I traveled the road to good health, I never stopped eating meat, but I changed my outlook and learned to appreciate simply prepared meals. It goes along with the idea that eating whole foods, or foods as close as possible to their natural state, is best. Roasted chicken, grilled pork chops, and seared steak. I tend to stay away from sauces and complicated ingredients when I cook meat and poultry, savoring the intrinsic flavors of the protein. I also eat less meat than I used to, having learned to appreciate vegetarian and fish main courses more than ever. I don't miss meat, but when I eat it, I am a very happy man! If you like meat—and I do—nothing alleviates certain cravings like a big, juicy steak, thick pork chop, or grilled butterflied leg of lamb. Try the Grilled Hanger Steak with Slow-Roasted Tomatoes and Watercress on page 179 or the Pork Chops with Cilantro–Pumpkin Seed Pesto on page 168 and you will quickly see what I mean.

This is because without protein you will never feel satisfied after a meal. More importantly, protein cannot be ignored for good health.

If you include meat in your diet, you won't be able to overlook it. I like to eat light proteins in the evening (chicken, turkey, and fish) and save the heavier ones (beef, pork, and lamb) for earlier in the day. This seems upside down, since most folks eat their "main" meal well into the evening, but consider how our forefathers lived. They came in from the fields to eat a hearty lunch and, after the day's chores were done, ate something light and fell into bed. So, if beef is on the menu, I try to eat it early in the evening or for lunch so that my body has ample time to metabolize it before I turn in. As a southerner, I love pork and especially appreciate ham. I'm not talking about the canned ham from the supermarket, but the artisanal product—such as Colonel Bill Newsom's Kentucky Country Ham, which is carefully aged and treated so it's full of wonderful flavor, and only a few delightfully salty, dry slices are needed to satisfy. Not everyone likes Smithfield-style hams when they first taste them, and I agree they are an acquired taste. Most Americans are far more familiar with cured, baked ham, which is what we buy at the deli counter and prepare for Easter dinner. When you are in the market for this kind of ham, buy it from a reputable butcher or market and go for the best you can find and afford.

There is a lot written about free-range chickens, grass-fed beef, and organic everything. I grew up on a farm in northern Florida, and our beef was grass fed because we couldn't afford to feed it any other way. Consequently, the flavor of today's much-heralded grass-fed meat is familiar to me. I like the idea that the animals from these farms are treated more humanely than others and I absolutely don't like the idea of "factory farms." I also try to buy organic poultry whenever I can. Its flavor is better. I appreciate the fact that these animals are not pumped full of hormones and antibiotics. I don't need those in my body. In the end, whatever your choice for meat, eat it in moderation, enjoy it fully, and appreciate the diversity it lends to meals.

Curried Pork Shoulder with Brown Rice and Mustard Greens ❋ 148

Barbecue Chicken Thighs with Sweet Potato Salad ❋ 150

Lemon-Roasted Chicken with Banana Peppers ❋ 152

Garlic-Braised Chicken Thighs with Quinoa ❋ 154

Kale-Stuffed Turkey Meat Loaf with Tomato-Caper Sauce ❋ 156

Herb-and-Mustard-Crusted Pork Tenderloin with Roasted Peaches ❋ 158

Unfried Chicken with Roasted Brussels Sprouts ❋ 160

Lamb Kabobs with Cucumber Raita ❋ 162

Skirt Steak with Chimichurri and Roasted Fingerling Potatoes ❋ 166

Pork Chops with Cilantro–Pumpkin Seed Pesto ❋ 168

Grilled Hanger Steak with Slow-Roasted Tomatoes and Watercress ❋ 170

Curried Pork Shoulder with Brown Rice and Mustard Greens

~~~~~~

This is one of those meals that says "fall"—one of my favorite seasons in Chicago, my adopted city. The lake shines bright blue, the air is crisp, and fresh mustard greens appear at the farmer's markets. Like many slow-cooked stews, this one is just as good or better the day after it's made.

Serves 8

For the pork:
1 boneless pork shoulder roast, about 2½ pounds
2 tablespoons low-sodium soy sauce
2 tablespoons curry powder
½ teaspoon cayenne
Salt
1 tablespoon canola oil
1 large onion, chopped
1 cup chopped carrots
¼ cup minced fresh ginger
4 garlic cloves, chopped
4 to 5 cups low-sodium chicken stock or water

For the rice:
3 cups low-sodium chicken stock or water
1½ cups brown rice

For the mustard greens:
6 ounces mustard greens, coarsely chopped

For the garnish:
½ cup loosely packed cilantro leaves
2 limes, quartered

METHOD To prepare the pork: Preheat the oven to 250°F.

Cut the pork shoulder into 1-inch cubes and place in a large mixing bowl. Add the soy sauce, curry powder, and cayenne and mix until thoroughly combined. Season with salt.

In a large Dutch oven or braising pan, warm the canola oil over medium-high heat. Add the pork pieces to the pan and sear over high heat for 5 to 7 minutes. Temporarily remove the pork from the pan. Add the onion, carrots, ginger, and garlic to the pan and cook for 5 to 7 minutes or until the vegetables begin to caramelize. Return the pork to the pan. Add the stock to the pan and bring to a simmer. Reduce the heat to a very low simmer, cover, and cook for 4 hours or until the pork is very tender and can be pulled apart with a fork.

To prepare the rice: Place the chicken stock and rice in a medium saucepan and bring to a boil over medium-high heat. Reduce to a low simmer. Cover the pot, leaving the lid ajar. Slowly simmer the rice for 40 to 45 minutes or until just cooked. Remove from the heat and fluff with a fork.

To prepare the mustard greens: In a medium saucepan, bring 1 inch of water to a simmer, add the mustard greens, and cover. Cook the mustard greens over medium heat for 2 to 3 minutes or until they are just wilted. Remove from the heat.

ASSEMBLY Divide the rice among the serving plates and top with the mustard greens. Spoon the curried pork shoulder (along with the vegetables and cooking liquid) over the rice and mustard greens. Garnish with the cilantro leaves and lime.

Per serving: 422 calories • 13 g fat • 4 g sat fat • 92 mg chol • 340 mg sodium • 39 g carb • 3 g sugar • 5 g fiber • 37 g protein • 78 mg calcium

Barbecue Chicken Thighs with
Sweet Potato Salad

~~~~~~

Chicken thighs are too often overlooked by home cooks, who tend to prefer white-meat chicken breasts, but the thighs are full flavored and often less expensive, too. Try them coated with this slightly spicy barbecue sauce and then grilled to perfection. The sweet potato salad is a delicious accompaniment. If you want to make the sauce ahead of time, it keeps in the refrigerator for up to a week.

Serves 6

For the sweet potato salad:
4 cups medium-diced sweet potato
½ cup nonfat Greek yogurt
½ cup chopped cilantro
2 tablespoons fresh lime juice
1 tablespoon fresh lemon juice
1 teaspoon ground cumin
½ cup minced red onion
2 celery stalks, peeled and thinly sliced
1 jalapeno pepper, seeded and minced
Salt

For the barbecue sauce:
8 ounces jarred or canned stewed tomatoes
¼ cup orange juice
2 tablespoons cider vinegar
1 tablespoon Worcestershire sauce
1 tablespoon Dijon mustard
1 tablespoon honey
1 serrano chili, cut in half
½ teaspoon smoked paprika

For the chicken thighs:
12 skinless and boneless chicken thighs

For the garnish:
3 green onions, chopped

METHOD **To prepare the sweet potato salad:** Place the sweet potatoes in a large saucepan and cover with water. Bring to a boil, then immediately reduce to a simmer. Cook the potatoes for 15 to 20 minutes or until fork tender. Drain the potatoes, place in a large mixing bowl, and cool to room temperature.

In a small mixing bowl, combine the yogurt, cilantro, lime juice, lemon juice, and cumin. Add the red onion, celery, jalapeno pepper, and the yogurt mixture to the sweet potatoes. Toss until combined. Cover and refrigerate for 1 hour. Season with salt after it chills.

To prepare the barbecue sauce: In a medium saucepan, combine the tomatoes, orange juice, cider vinegar, Worcestershire sauce, Dijon mustard, honey, chili, and paprika. Bring to a simmer over medium heat and slowly simmer for 15 minutes. Remove the chili from the pot and discard. Puree the barbecue sauce with a handheld immersion blender or in a blender. Refrigerate until ready to use.

To prepare the chicken thighs: Place the chicken thighs in a 1-gallon plastic bag with half the barbecue sauce. Seal the bag and move the chicken around in the bag so that it is coated with the sauce. Refrigerate for 1 hour.

Preheat a grill to moderate heat.

Place the chicken thighs on the grill over moderate heat and cook for 6 to 8 minutes on each side or until done. Brush with additional barbecue sauce during the final minutes of cooking.

ASSEMBLY Place two barbecued chicken thighs on each plate and divide the Sweet Potato Salad among the 6 serving plates. Sprinkle the chopped green onions over the chicken and Sweet Potato Salad.

Per serving: 349 calories • 12 g fat • 3 g sat fat • 99 mg chol • 343 mg sodium • 30 g carb • 10 g sugar • 4 g fiber • 31 g protein • 85 mg calcium

$\mathcal{L}$emon-Roasted Chicken
with Banana Peppers

~~~~~~

$\mathbf{A}$ whole roasted chicken is not only one of the most comforting and tender ways to serve chicken—it's easy, too. This one is roasted with mild banana peppers, onions, and zucchini, so you don't have to worry too much about what to serve alongside the chicken. Stick with these veggies and perhaps a green salad. You're done!

Serves 6

For the chicken:
1 whole roasting chicken (4½ pounds)
Salt
1 teaspoon smoked paprika
2 lemons, sliced into ¼-inch-thick pieces
8 garlic cloves, peeled and smashed
4 banana peppers, cut into ½-inch-thick pieces
2 Vidalia onions, each cut into 8 pieces
2 zucchini, sliced into ½-inch-thick rounds
1 cup low-sodium chicken stock or water

For the garnish:
8 basil leaves, chopped

METHOD Preheat the oven to 425°F.

Season the chicken with salt and the smoked paprika. Be sure to season the chicken's cavity with a little salt, then put 3 lemon slices inside the chicken cavity.

In a large roasting pan, place the remaining lemon slices, garlic, banana peppers, onions, and zucchini. Sit the seasoned chicken on top of the vegetables. Pour the chicken stock in the roasting pan around but not over the chicken.

Place the pan in the oven and roast the chicken for 1 hour and 10 minutes or until the thickest part of the thigh registers 160°F on an instant-read thermometer and the juices run clear.

Remove from the oven and let rest for 15 minutes before serving.

ASSEMBLY Carve the chicken and place on a serving platter with the vegetables. Sprinkle with the chopped basil. Spoon any cooking juices that remain in the pan over the vegetables.

Per serving: 269 calories • 6 g fat • 1 g sat fat • 114 mg chol • 159 mg sodium • 18 g carb • 7 g sugar • 5 g fiber • 39 g protein • 88 mg calcium

Protein Rules!

Plain and simple, we need protein to stay alive. While protein is essential for everyone, it's particularly important for children, adolescents, and pregnant women. Luckily, for most of us living in the United States and other developed countries, getting enough protein is not much of a problem. It's found in meat, fish, and poultry. It's also in dairy products, eggs, legumes, nuts, and soy.

The amino acids in protein are not stored in the body and so must be replaced regularly to repair cells and build new ones. Amino acids are truly the building blocks of life.

For those of us concerned about eating healthfully and living well, it's a good idea to think about the other aspects of a high-protein meal. Sure, a T-bone steak has a lot of protein, but it is also marbled with saturated fat. Not

good! Have that steak very rarely (and when you do, enjoy every bite!). Instead, get your protein from chicken and fish, both of which are leaner and therefore better for you.

Vegetarians can count on getting enough protein from dairy products, eggs, soy, nuts, and legumes. Vegans have to be a little more diligent, as they eschew eggs and dairy. Regardless of your dietary convictions, it's crucial to get enough protein.

What happens if we don't? We lose muscle mass, our immune systems weaken, and eventually, so do our hearts and respiratory systems. Doesn't sound good, does it?

It's not!

However, as I said earlier, it's pretty easy to get enough protein if you eat sensibly. ❋

Garlic-Braised Chicken Thighs with Quinoa

I like to braise chicken thighs because they, unlike the drier breasts, stay moist during the relatively long simmer. Served on top of quinoa with the succulent braising vegetables and juices, they make a mouth-watering meal.

Serves 4

For the chicken:
1 tablespoon canola oil
8 skinless and boneless chicken thighs
8 cloves garlic, peeled and smashed
1 red onion, peeled and coarsely chopped
2 cups low-sodium chicken stock or water
2 red bell peppers, seeded and cut into 1-inch pieces
1 lemon, cut into eighths
1 tablespoon chopped fresh oregano
Salt and freshly ground black pepper

For the quinoa:
1 cup quinoa, rinsed
1 tablespoon extra-virgin olive oil
1 tablespoon lemon juice
2 tablespoons chopped flat-leaf parsley
Salt and freshly ground black pepper

METHOD **To prepare the chicken thighs:** Heat the oil in a Dutch oven over medium-high heat and brown the chicken, 2 to 3 minutes on each side. Transfer to a plate. Add the garlic and onion to the pot and cook until golden, about 5 minutes. Return the chicken thighs to the pot. Add the stock or water, bell peppers, lemon, and oregano and bring to a boil. Reduce to a slow simmer and cover, leaving the lid slightly ajar. Cook for about 40 minutes or until the chicken is cooked through. Season to taste with salt and pepper.

To prepare the quinoa: Place the quinoa in a medium saucepan and cover with 2 cups cold water. Bring to a boil and immediately reduce to a simmer. Cover, leaving the lid slightly ajar. Continue to cook over low heat for 15 to 20 minutes or until the quinoa is puffed and you see a little white ring release from the quinoa germ. Remove from the heat and fold in the olive oil, lemon juice, and parsley. Season with salt and pepper.

ASSEMBLY Divide the quinoa among 4 shallow serving bowls and top with two chicken thighs and some of the braising vegetables. Spoon any liquid that remains in the pot over the chicken.

Per serving: 491 calories • 22 g fat • 4 g sat fat • 99 mg chol • 118 mg sodium • 40 g carb • 4 g sugar • 6 g fiber • 36 g protein • 80 mg calcium

Kale-Stuffed Turkey Meat Loaf with Tomato-Caper Sauce

~~~~~~

If there are quintessential comfort foods, meat loaf might top the list. I know it is certainly in my top five. I have come up with a version that is more loaf than meat and packed with health-giving vegetables. It takes a little effort to stuff and roll the meat loaf, and I suggest a homemade tomato sauce to replace sugary ketchup. The result? Fantastic! And how about some meat loaf sandwiches tomorrow?

Serves 8

For the tomato-caper sauce:
2 tablespoons extra-virgin olive oil
4 cloves garlic, minced
1 medium yellow onion, chopped
2 18-ounce jars or cans chopped tomatoes
¼ cup chopped fresh basil
3 tablespoons capers, rinsed
1 tablespoon balsamic vinegar
Salt

For the stuffing:
1 tablespoon extra-virgin olive oil
1 large yellow onion, chopped
½ pound fresh kale, thick stems removed and remaining leaves
    chopped
⅓ cup grated pecorino Romano cheese
1 tablespoon balsamic vinegar

For the meat loaf:
2 pounds ground turkey breast
1 large egg
1 large egg white
1 cup whole wheat panko bread crumbs
2 tablespoons Dijon mustard
1 tablespoon dried oregano
1 tablespoon Worcestershire sauce
Salt and freshly ground black pepper

METHOD To prepare the sauce: Place the olive oil in a medium sauce-pan and warm over medium heat. Add the garlic and onion to the pan and cook over medium-high heat for 6 to 8 minutes or until the onion is translucent. If the garlic appears to burn, reduce the heat a little. Add the tomatoes and bring to a simmer. Continue to simmer over low heat for 30 minutes. Add the basil, capers, and vinegar and season with salt. Reheat prior to serving.

To prepare the stuffing: Place the olive oil in a preheated large sauté pan. Add the onion and cook over medium-high heat for 5 minutes. Add the kale and ½ cup water to the pan. Cover and cook the kale and onions for 2 minutes. Remove the lid and continue to cook the kale until it has wilted. Remove from the heat and stir in the cheese and vinegar. Cool the kale to room temperature.

To prepare the meat loaf: Preheat the oven to 350°F.

In a large mixing bowl, combine the ground turkey, egg, egg white, bread crumbs, Dijon mustard, oregano, and Worcestershire sauce. Season with salt and pepper.

Lay a 12-inch-long piece of plastic wrap on the counter. Evenly spread the ground turkey mixture on the plastic wrap, leaving a 1-inch border on all sides. Spread the kale mixture down the middle of the ground turkey, leaving a 1-inch border.

Lift the plastic wrap along the long side facing you and roll the meat and stuffing like a jelly roll until it forms a long log. Make sure you pull the plastic wrap away as you roll up the log, as the plastic will be discarded prior to baking.

Carefully transfer the stuffed meat loaf to a roasting pan. Bake the meat loaf, uncovered, for 45 minutes. Pour half the tomato sauce over the meat loaf. Continue to cook for 15 minutes more or until it reaches an internal temperature of 160°F on an instant-read thermometer.

Remove the meat loaf from the oven and let it rest for 15 minutes.

ASSEMBLY Slice the meat loaf into 1-inch-thick slices and shingle on a serving platter. Pour the remaining tomato sauce over the meat loaf.

Per serving: 313 calories • 9 g fat • 2 g sat fat • 77 mg chol • 711 mg sodium • 26 g carb • 6 g sugar • 4 g fiber • 36 g protein • 142 mg calcium

Herb-and-Mustard-Crusted Pork Tenderloin
with Roasted Peaches

~~~~~~

Pork and peaches. What a team. You may not have thought of this pairing, but if you like pork with apples or pears, you'll love it with sweet, juicy peaches. Roasting the fruit just makes it sweeter. Once you try it alongside the pork, you'll be a convert.

Serves 4

For the pork:
1 pork tenderloin
Salt and freshly ground black pepper
2 tablespoons Dijon mustard
2 tablespoons herbes de Provence

For the peaches:
3 peaches
1 tablespoon extra-virgin olive oil
1 sprig rosemary

METHOD **To prepare the pork:** Preheat the oven to 425°F.

Season the pork on all sides with salt and pepper. Rub the mustard completely over the pork and sprinkle it with the herbes de Provence. Place in a roasting pan and roast for 40 to 45 minutes or until the pork reaches an internal temperature of 140°F on an instant-read thermometer. Remove from the oven and let rest for 15 minutes before slicing into ½-inch-thick pieces.

To prepare the peaches: Preheat the oven to 425°F.

Blanch the peaches in boiling water for 1 minute and immediately shock in a bowl of ice water. Remove and discard the skins. Cut the peaches into eighths. Place the peach slices in an ovenproof pan and drizzle the olive oil over them. Add the rosemary sprig. Cover the pan and roast in the oven for 15 minutes or until the peaches are tender. Discard the rosemary sprig.

ASSEMBLY Divide the pork among 4 serving plates and spoon the roasted peaches over the top.

Per serving: 328 calories • 9 g fat • 2 g sat fat • 147 mg chol • 300 mg sodium • 12 g carb • 9 g sugar • 2 g fiber • 49 g protein • 18 mg calcium

Forget About Low Fat

If the food you eat is low in fat, you won't get fat. Makes sense, right? Not necessarily. I am not saying that you should never buy low-fat or nonfat foods, because you should (think about skim milk and nonfat yogurt). Yet, as with so much in life, when it comes to fat, moderation is the name of the game. Better still is to learn about "good" and "bad" fats, and avoid the latter and eat the former—in moderation.

Polyunsaturated fats, found in soy and soy oil, corn oil, walnuts, and sesame seeds, are good for you. They improve blood cholesterol levels, so you are less likely to develop heart disease, and they also might decrease the chance of developing type 2 diabetes. Omega-3 fatty acids are found in polyunsaturated fats, most often in oily fish such as salmon, tuna, and sardines but also in flaxseeds, flaxseed oil, and other foods. Omega-3s have been shown to reduce the risk of coronary artery disease and could lower your blood pressure. For this reason, many people take fish oil supplements to boost their intake of omega-3 fatty acids.

Monounsaturated fats, found in extra-virgin olive oil, canola oil, avocados, nuts, and peanut butter, help stabilize your cholesterol levels. They also help regulate blood sugar levels, which is beneficial if you suffer from type 2 diabetes. Monounsaturated fats are considered a little more beneficial than polyunsaturated, although a balanced and varied diet is likely to supply a combination of both.

Saturated fats, such as butter, milk, cheese, and animal fat, actually raise blood cholesterol levels, both HDL and LDL. This is not good and can lead to cardiovascular disease and type 2 diabetes, as well as other health problems.

Still, you need dietary fat in your diet, and it's better to eat a little saturated fat, say a pat of butter or small scoop of ice cream, than to compensate with soda, candy, or another type of carbohydrate that is nothing but empty calories.

Fat—polyunsaturated, monounsaturated, and saturated—should never make up more than 25 to 35 percent of your daily diet (and saturated fat should not be more than 10 percent of your overall intake in a day).

Don't want to do the math? Eat vegetable fat. While you need some each day, don't eat too much. And stay away from animal fat, although a little won't hurt you. ※

$\mathcal{U}$nfried Chicken with Roasted Brussels Sprouts

W ith tongue in cheek, I call this chicken "unfried." That's because I am well known for fried chicken, which may be the crown jewel of southern cooking but is a dish I avoid these days. I like unfried chicken just as much. The chicken is soaked in tangy buttermilk and then coated with flavorful breading, just like fried chicken. The difference is that it's baked. This dish was on the menu at LYFE Kitchen. I first prepared it when Oprah's movie *Beloved* opened. One of the many lessons I learned from Oprah is to offer people a choice at meals, and one of those choices should be a healthy one. To this day I honor that lesson in my home and my restaurants.

Serves 4

For the chicken:
1 cup buttermilk
1 tablespoon Louisiana Hot Sauce or another hot sauce
4 skinless and boneless chicken breasts, cut in half
1½ cups multigrain or whole wheat panko bread crumbs
3 tablespoons grated Parmesan cheese
2 teaspoons ground black pepper
1 teaspoon cayenne
1½ teaspoons onion powder
1½ teaspoons garlic powder
1 teaspoon paprika

For the brussels sprouts:
16 brussels sprouts, cut in half
1½ tablespoons extra-virgin olive oil
Salt and freshly ground black pepper

For the garnish:
1 lemon, quartered

METHOD **To prepare the chicken:** Preheat the oven to 400°F.

In a mixing bowl, mix the buttermilk and hot sauce. Submerge the chicken pieces in the buttermilk and soak in the refrigerator for at least 1 hour but no more than 24 hours.

In a gallon-size plastic bag, combine the bread crumbs, Parmesan, black pepper, cayenne, onion powder, garlic powder, and paprika. Seal the bag and shake until well mixed.

Remove the chicken from the buttermilk and transfer directly to the bag with the bread crumb mixture. Shake the bag until the chicken breasts are evenly coated with the bread crumbs. Remove the chicken breasts from the bag and lay flat on a nonstick baking sheet. Refrigerate, uncovered, for 30 minutes.

Bake the chicken for 20 to 25 minutes or until just cooked through.

To prepare the brussels sprouts: Preheat the oven to 400°F.

Place brussels sprouts in a medium mixing bowl, toss with the olive oil, and season with salt and pepper. Spread the brussels sprouts in a medium ovenproof baking dish and roast for 20 minutes or until caramelized and tender.

ASSEMBLY Divide the chicken and brussels sprouts among 4 serving plates, and squeeze the lemon over the chicken.

Per serving: 427 calories • 12 g fat • 3 g sat fat • 79 mg chol • 349 mg sodium • 45 g carb • 6 g sugar • 9 g fiber • 40 g protein • 185 mg calcium

$\mathcal{L}$amb Kabobs with Cucumber Raita

$\mathcal{B}$ecause lamb is commonly served in India with a cooling yogurt-based condiment called raita, I decided to follow suit. And then I jumped continents to serve this with quinoa, an ancient Peruvian crop that is a great favorite with modern-day cooks, including me.

Serves 4 to 6

For the quinoa:
1 cup quinoa, rinsed
Salt
1 tablespoon fresh lemon juice
1 tablespoon extra-virgin olive oil
2 tablespoons chopped flat-leaf parsley

For the raita:
12 ounces nonfat Greek yogurt
⅓ cup diced, peeled, and seeded cucumber
3 tablespoons chopped fresh mint leaves
1½ tablespoons fresh lemon juice
1 large garlic clove, minced
Salt

For the lamb:
1 pound boneless leg of lamb, trimmed and cut into 1-inch pieces
1 tablespoon curry powder
2 tablespoons extra-virgin olive oil
Salt
16 grape or cherry tomatoes
1 yellow bell pepper, seeded and cut into 1-inch pieces
8 10-inch bamboo skewers, soaked in water

METHOD **To prepare the quinoa:** Place the quinoa in a medium saucepan. Cover with 2 cups cold water and add a pinch of salt. Cover the pan and bring to a boil. As soon as it begins to boil, reduce the heat to a simmer and set the lid slightly ajar to prevent boiling over. Simmer the quinoa for 15 to 20 minutes or until the liquid has been fully absorbed. You should see a little white ring release from the quinoa germ. Remove from heat, fluff with a fork, and stir in the lemon juice, olive oil, and parsley.

To prepare the raita: In a small mixing bowl, combine the yogurt, cucumber, mint, lemon juice, and garlic. Mix with a wooden spoon until fully incorporated. Season with salt. Cover and refrigerate until ready to use.

To prepare the lamb: Preheat a grill to moderate heat.

In a medium mixing bowl, combine the lamb, curry powder, and 1 tablespoon of the olive oil. Season with salt.

In a separate mixing bowl, combine the tomatoes and bell pepper. Toss with the remaining 1 tablespoon extra-virgin olive oil and season with salt. Thread the lamb, bell pepper, and tomatoes alternately onto the skewers.

Place the prepared kabobs on the grill and cook for 5 minutes on each side or until cooked.

ASSEMBLY Spoon some quinoa on each plate, top with two lamb kabobs, and spoon some raita over the lamb. Sprinkle with additional chopped mint, if desired.

Per serving: 478 calories • 9 g fat • 4 g sat fat • 73 mg chol • 133 mg sodium • 39 g carb • 7 g sugar • 5 g fiber • 38 g protein • 112 mg calcium

Conquering Restaurants

You think you have trouble in restaurants? Try being a chef! I have learned a thing or two over the past couple of years about surviving restaurant food and its temptations and have assembled a dozen tips. Some are obvious—no doubt you have heard them before—and some may be new to you. All make perfect sense and have saved me a few pounds and more than a few sleepless nights brought on by rich, heavy food.

First a look behind the scenes, in the restaurant kitchens. I travel a lot while visiting my five restaurants, which are in New York, Washington, Atlanta, Chicago, and California. When I began the journey to reclaim my health and lose weight, all the chefs who worked at the restaurants were supportive. They prepared healthful salads and soups for me to nosh on, and when we tasted new menu items, they understood when I took only a bite. I felt bad about this; a young chef might have toiled for hours to showcase his creation for me, but I had to stand firm. And you know what? I learned that a bite or two gave me a very good idea of the value of any given dish. As a side note, many of these cooks started joining me at the gym. When they saw the progress I was making and took note of how much better I felt, they happily joined in. The result? We are a more cheerful and productive team.

Now for the twelve tips. When you are a guest at a restaurant, you won't want to take only a bite. Going out to eat is a treat. We don't have to cook, we can sit back and relax as someone else does the work, and best of all, we can visit with family and friends in a pleasant environment. Some restaurants are quiet and serene, others are a little more boisterous and "happening," but all share a desire to make their customers happy with good food and service. But because they are all about food and drink, they can be a minefield for people watching their weight and their health. Behold! the baker's dozen:

1. Don't arrive at the restaurant ravenous. Eat a few apple slices, a carrot, or a handful of nuts before you leave home or the office to ensure you won't devour the bread basket as soon as you sit down.

2. Order a salad as a first course, dressing on the side. Choose the salad with the most vegetables and least amount of cheese and croutons. Ask for a light dressing (vinaigrette) on the side, rather than a gloppy creamy dressing. If you are up for it, a lot of restaurants are happy to supply you with cruets of olive oil and vinegar so that you can make your own dressing at the table.

3. Order off the menu even if there is a buffet. It's far easier to control portion sizes and steer clear of "danger" foods if you do.

4. Order an appetizer or side dish as an entrée. When you do this, the portion will be smaller than an entrée serving and you can indulge in some very special treats.

5. Order grilled, broiled, or steamed fish, or grilled or broiled chicken or red meat. You want to steer clear of heavy sauces and an overload of ingredients.

6. If you must have pasta (and sometimes you must!), order whole wheat pasta, if

possible, and then stick with simple tomato sauces. Avoid cream and cheese-laden toppings.

7. Stop eating when your hunger is satisfied. Drink some water, sit back and smile at your fellow diners, and enjoy the conversation rather than the food. There is no reason to clean your plate.

8. Take home what you don't eat. Believe me, restaurants are only too happy to provide to-go boxes or pack up your food for transport.

9. Split an entrée with another diner. Most kitchens will prepare two plates before they bring out the food.

10. Order a single dessert for the table and ask for forks for everyone.

11. If others are ordering their own desserts, ask for a bowl of fruit or a simple sorbet.

12. Drink water rather than alcohol. Or switch to water after a glass of wine or a single cocktail. ❄

Skirt Steak with Chimichurri and Roasted Fingerling Potatoes

~~~~~~

Just because you're eating healthfully, that's no reason to completely forgo steak and potatoes. Skirt steak is especially flavorful and is even better when lightly marinated. If you have a butcher, ask for a skirt steak from the outside of the cut, which will be more tender and juicy than a skirt steak from the inside of the cut. Intense, herbaceous chimichurri has to be tasted to be believed. Invented in Argentina, where they love their steak, it's absolutely delicious, and yet a little goes a long way.

Serves 4

For the chimichurri:
1 cup chopped cilantro
1½ cups chopped flat-leaf parsley
⅓ cup extra-virgin olive oil
2 garlic cloves, chopped
3 tablespoons fresh lime juice
1 tablespoon fresh lemon juice
1 tablespoon apple cider vinegar
Salt

For the fingerling potatoes:
12 medium fingerling potatoes, washed
2 teaspoons extra-virgin olive oil
Salt and freshly ground black pepper

For the skirt steak:
16 ounces skirt steak
1 tablespoon balsamic vinegar
1 tablespoon extra-virgin olive oil
Salt and freshly ground black pepper

METHOD To prepare the chimichurri: Place the cilantro, parsley, oil, garlic, lime juice, lemon juice, and apple cider vinegar in a blender. Pulse to combine. Season with salt.

To prepare the potatoes and skirt steak: Preheat a grill to moderate heat.

Lay a large piece of aluminum foil flat on the counter. Place the fingerling potatoes on the foil. Drizzle the olive oil over the potatoes and season with salt and pepper. Seal up the aluminum foil, making sure the potatoes are well wrapped. Place on the grill over moderate heat or on a warming rack above the grill. Cook for 20 minutes or until just cooked.

Rub the skirt steak with the balsamic vinegar and olive oil and season with salt and pepper. Place the steak on the grill and cook for 5 to 8 minutes on each side or to desired doneness. (The steak can be marinated up to a day ahead in a sealed plastic bag.)

Remove the steak from the grill and transfer to a cutting board. Let the steak rest for 5 minutes before slicing into ½-inch-thick slices across the grain.

ASSEMBLY Arrange 3 potatoes on each plate alongside some of the sliced steak. Spoon 2 to 3 tablespoons of the chimichurri over the steak and potatoes.

Per serving: 594 calories • 34 g fat • 7 g sat fat • 65 mg chol • 106 mg sodium • 45 g carb • 4 g sugar • 5 g fiber • 36 g protein • 72 mg calcium

Pork Chops with
Cilantro–Pumpkin Seed Pesto

Broiled pork chops topped with this boldly flavored pesto make a terrific meal. You'll want to add a side dish or green salad, but the star of the show will be the chops. I like to make pesto with ingredients other than the traditional basil and Parmesan cheese. This one is made with pumpkin seeds and cilantro. Wonderful.

Serves 4

For the pesto:
½ cup shelled pumpkin seeds (pepitos), toasted
½ cup firmly packed cilantro leaves
2 cloves garlic, minced
4 tablespoons extra-virgin olive oil
2 tablespoons fresh lime juice
Salt

For the pork chops:
4 pork chops, on the bone
Salt and freshly ground black pepper

For the garnish:
1 lime, quartered

METHOD To prepare the pesto: In the bowl of a food processor fitted with a metal blade, mix the pumpkin seeds, cilantro leaves, garlic, oil, and lime juice. Puree until all the ingredients are fully incorporated and the mixture is finely ground. Season to taste with salt.

To prepare the pork chops: Preheat the broiler.

Season the pork chops with salt and pepper and place on the broiler pan rack. Broil the pork chops for 5 to 6 minutes on each side or until just cooked through. The internal temperature should be 160°F on an instant-read thermometer.

ASSEMBLY Place a pork chop on each plate and spoon the pesto over the pork chops. Squeeze lime juice over the pesto and pork chop.

Per serving: 248 calories • 23 g fat • 4 g sat fat • 12 mg chol • 12 mg sodium • 6 g carb • 1 g sugar • 1 g fiber • 8 g protein • 20 mg calcium

I generally prefer a thick-cut pork chop; they tend to cook up nicer while staying moist. Berkshire pork chops are a special treat. They are prized for their juiciness, flavor, and tenderness. They are generally higher in fat, which makes them suitable for high-temperature cooking. If you do get your hand on a Berkshire pork chop, they are best cooked with a little pink remaining in the flesh.

Grilled Hanger Steak with
Slow-Roasted Tomatoes and Watercress

~~~~~~

Hanger steak is a darling of restaurant chefs. Since it's on the menu at Art and Soul, I must plead guilty to a weakness for this treat. Time was when it was considered too homely to sell to the general public, but its rich flavor, thickness, and juiciness belie its lumpy appearance, and nowadays everyone loves it. I marinate hangers in mellow Banyuls vinegar, which is made from sweet grenache grapes and then aged. If you can't find this particular vinegar, substitute sherry or red wine vinegar.

Serves 4

For the tomatoes:
24 cherry tomatoes
6 cloves garlic, smashed
2 tablespoons fresh lemon juice
2 sprigs thyme
2 tablespoons extra-virgin olive oil

For the steak:
24 ounces hanger steak
1 tablespoon Banyuls vinegar
1 tablespoon extra-virgin olive oil
Salt and freshly ground black pepper

For the watercress:
4 cups watercress, thick stems discarded
1 teaspoon Banyuls vinegar
1 tablespoon extra-virgin olive oil
Salt and freshly ground black pepper

METHOD To prepare the tomatoes: Preheat the oven to 250°F.

Score the tops of the tomatoes with a knife. Place the tomatoes, garlic cloves, lemon juice, thyme, and olive oil in a small ovenproof pan (you do not want lots of extra room in the pan). Cover the pan with aluminum foil. Slowly roast the tomatoes in the oven for 2 hours or until the skins are pulling away. Discard the thyme sprigs and tomato skins.

To prepare the steak: Place the steak in a plastic bag and add the vinegar and olive oil. Seal the bag tightly and move the steak around to ensure it is coated with the vinegar and oil. Refrigerate for 1 hour.

Preheat a grill to moderate heat.

Remove the steak from the bag. Season with salt and generously with pepper. Cook for 7 to 8 minutes on each side or until medium-rare. Remove from the grill and let rest for 5 to 10 minutes before slicing into ½-inch-thick slices.

To prepare the watercress: Just prior to serving, place the watercress in a medium mixing bowl. Toss with the vinegar and olive oil, then season with salt and pepper.

ASSEMBLY Divide the tomatoes among 4 serving plates. Spoon any juices still in the pan and drizzle them over the tomatoes. Top with the sliced steak and watercress.

Per serving: 431 calories • 28 g fat • 7 g sat fat • 97 mg chol • 134 mg sodium • 7 g carb • 3 g sugar • 2 g fiber • 38 g protein • 74 mg calcium

10

Vegetable Side Dishes

Most of us eat vegetables as a side dish, an accent to the "main" event. Go for it! Cook a wide variety of vegetables and let your creativity have a field day when it comes to these gorgeous sides. Fill half your plate with them and be prepared to feel better. Have seconds. You won't overdo it when it comes to vegetables, particularly green veggies (and I include squash and carrots in this category). You have to be a little more restrained when it comes to grains and potatoes, even sweet potatoes, but that's okay.

For many home cooks, prepping vegetables is a turnoff. So much peeling, washing, chopping, steaming, blanching. Phew! Yes, it's true that many vegetables require a little time in the kitchen, but they also make perfect leftovers (make a lot when you cook them) and freeze beautifully (chop up more than you need and stash them in the freezer for later use). Vegetables are great for a late-night snack or to fill the hunger void at the end of the afternoon—easy to digest, bursting with vitamins, and a great source of fiber. Many chefs like them cooked al dente so they have a little crunch. I prefer mine cooked longer; slowly braised greens and long-simmered beans are divine, if you ask me. However you like them, eat them. You'll never be sorry you ate your vegetables!

Gingered Carrots ✳ 175

Creamy Polenta with Wild Mushrooms ✳ 176

Curried Quinoa ✳ 178

Nelson Mandela's Brown Basmati Rice with Spinach and Peas ✳ 179

Sweet Potato Salad with Cumin and Cilantro ✳ 181

Roasted Acorn Squash and Honey ✳ 182

Green Beans and Tomatoes ✳ 183

Pickled Red Beets with Goat Cheese ✳ 184

Cannellini Beans and Roasted Fennel ✳ 185

Roasted Leeks ✳ 186

Spinach Custard ✳ 187

Sugar Snap Peas with Lemon ✳ 188

Slow-Roasted Tomatoes ✳ 189

Field Pea and Hominy Succotash ✳ 190

Fava Bean, Radish, and Corn Salad ✳ 192

Grilled Radicchio ✳ 193

Braised Collard Greens with Smoked Turkey ✳ 194

Roasted Cauliflower with Pepperoncini ✳ 195

Art Smith's Healthy Comfort

Gingered Carrots

~~~~~~

I like to make this dish with real baby carrots that still have the greens attached. You may not be able to find them, so don't ignore this recipe if your supermarket has only plastic sacks of "baby carrots." These often are cut from larger carrots, but they still taste good, especially when cooked with ginger and cilantro. Farmer's markets are good places for the real thing, so check them out in the springtime—but eat these all year long.

Serves 4

1 pound baby carrots, peeled with the stem end attached
1 tablespoon canola oil
2 teaspoons minced fresh ginger
1 tablespoon chopped cilantro
1 tablespoon lemon juice
Salt and freshly ground black pepper

METHOD Place the carrots in the basket of a prepared stove-top steamer and steam them for 10 minutes or until tender. Remove from the steamer.

Place the canola oil in a preheated medium sauté pan. Add the ginger and cook over medium heat for 1 minute or until fragrant. Add the carrots to the pan and continue to cook for 2 minutes. Remove from the heat and toss with the cilantro and lemon juice, then season with salt and pepper.

ASSEMBLY Place the carrots in a serving dish and serve hot or at room temperature.

Per serving: 86 calories • 4 g fat • 0 g sat fat • 0 mg chol • 60 mg sodium • 13 g carb • 7 g sugar • 3 g fiber • 1 g protein • 27 mg calcium

Creamy Polenta with Wild Mushrooms

Mushrooms and polenta are a great team. Together they produce a side dish that is earthy, rich, and filling. What more could you want? Use your favorite mushrooms or those that are easy to find. If you can't come up with anything other than common white mushrooms, use them. Just don't miss this.

Serves 4

For the mushrooms:
4 teaspoons extra-virgin olive oil
1 shallot, minced
8 ounces wild mushrooms (cremini, oyster, shitake), cleaned and thinly
    sliced
Salt and freshly ground black pepper

For the polenta:
1 cup polenta
1 tablespoon extra-virgin olive oil
¼ cup grated Parmesan cheese
4 tablespoons chopped fresh basil
Salt and freshly ground black pepper

METHOD To prepare the mushrooms: Warm the olive oil in a preheated large sauté pan. Add the shallot and cook for 1 minute over medium heat. Add the mushrooms and continue to cook for 7 to 10 minutes or until the mushrooms are tender. Remove from the heat and season with salt and pepper.

To prepare the polenta: In a medium saucepan, bring 3 cups of water to a simmer, add the polenta, and whisk until there are no lumps. Cover with a lid and continue to cook over low heat for 20 minutes, stirring every 3 minutes or so. Be careful when you stir the polenta; it tends to spit out pieces of the very hot cornmeal.

Remove the polenta from the heat and stir in the olive oil, Parmesan cheese, and basil. Season with salt and pepper.

ASSEMBLY Pour the hot polenta into a serving dish and spoon the mushrooms over the polenta.

Per serving: 286 calories • 13 g fat • 3 g sat fat • 8 mg chol • 448 mg sodium • 35 g carb • 3 g sugar • 3 g fiber • 9 g protein • 140 mg calcium

I really enjoy the satisfying feeling of a warm spoonful of creamy polenta straight out of the pan. But for some reason I always make too much. The leftover polenta can be spread out into a small casserole dish and refrigerated. Once set you can cut the now firm polenta into squares, discs, or sticks that can easily be reheated and enjoyed with a poached or fried egg on top.

Curried Quinoa

As I've said before, I am crazy about quinoa, an ancient grain from South America that is becoming pretty well known here. Quinoa is actually a seed, but it cooks like a grain and as such is an important part of a healthful diet. Like grains, it is a slowly absorbed carb that tastes good and leaves you feeling satisfied. This recipe is as easy as can be. A little curry powder, a little lemon juice, a little olive oil, and you're all set.

Serves 4

1 cup quinoa, rinsed
1 teaspoon curry powder
1 tablespoon extra-virgin olive oil
1 tablespoon fresh lemon juice
2 tablespoons chopped flat-leaf parsley
Salt and freshly ground black pepper

METHOD Place the quinoa and curry powder in a medium saucepan and cover with 2 cups cold water. Bring to a boil and immediately reduce to a simmer. Cover, leaving the lid slightly ajar, and continue to cook over low heat for 15 to 20 minutes or until the quinoa is puffed and you see a little white ring release from the quinoa germ. Remove from the heat. Fold in the olive oil, lemon juice, and parsley, then season to taste with salt and pepper.

ASSEMBLY Place the quinoa in a serving bowl. The quinoa can be enjoyed hot, warm, or chilled.

Per serving: 190 calories • 6 g fat • 1 g sat fat • 0 mg chol • 3 mg sodium • 28 g carb • 0 g sugar • 3 g fiber • 6 g protein • 25 mg calcium

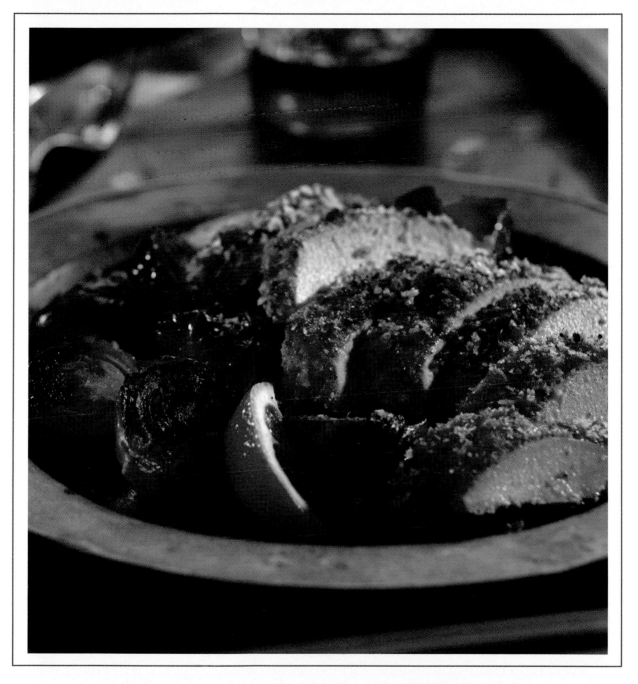

※ UNFRIED CHICKEN WITH ROASTED BRUSSELS SPROUTS (page 160) ※

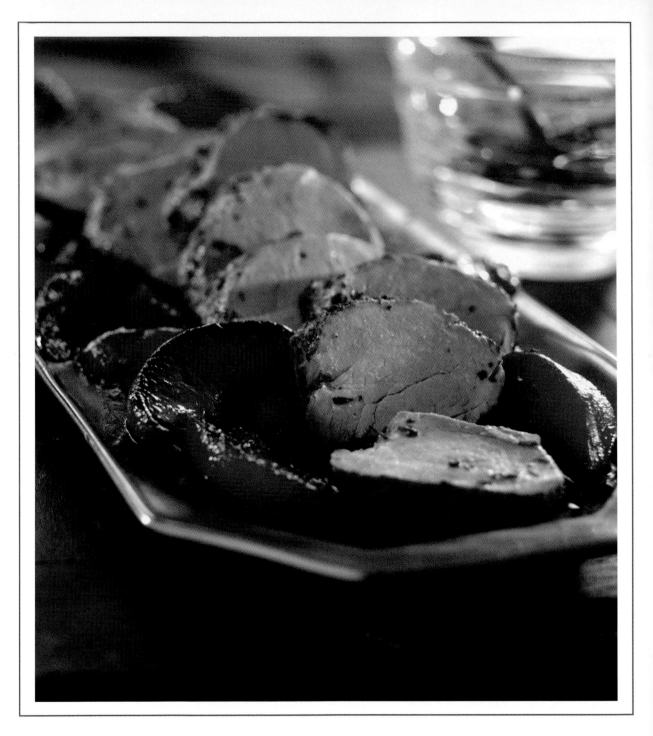

❋ HERB-AND-MUSTARD-CRUSTED PORK TENDERLOIN WITH ROASTED PEACHES (page 158) ❋

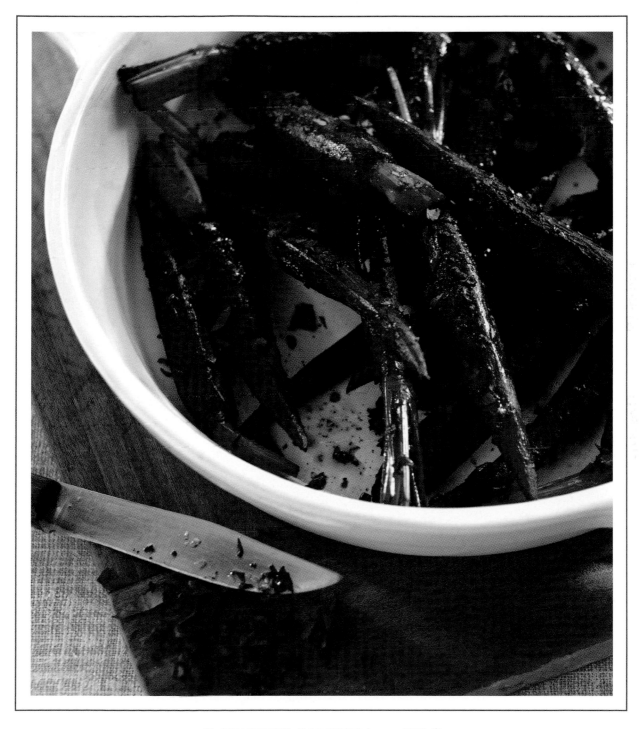

❋ GINGERED CARROTS (page 175) ❋

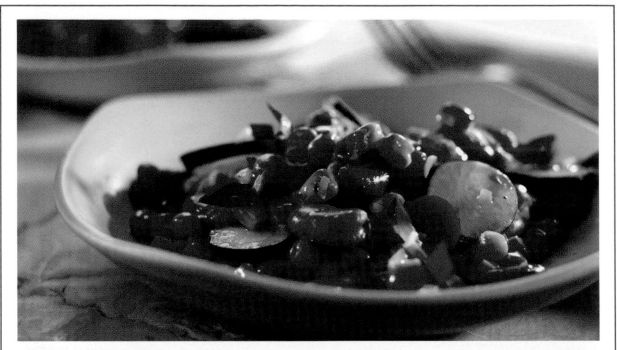

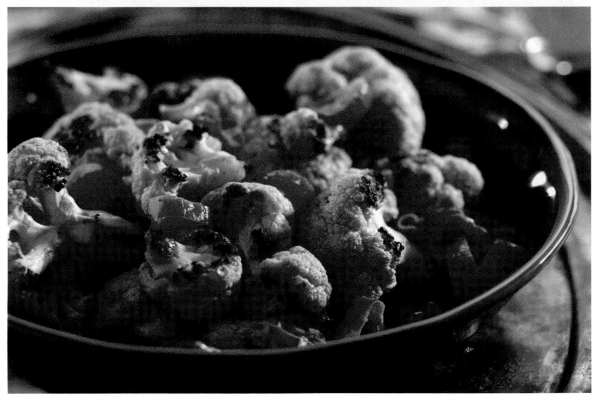

❋ *Top:* FAVA BEAN, RADISH, AND CORN SALAD (page 192) ❋
❋ *Bottom:* ROASTED CAULIFLOWER WITH PEPPERONCINI (page 195) ❋

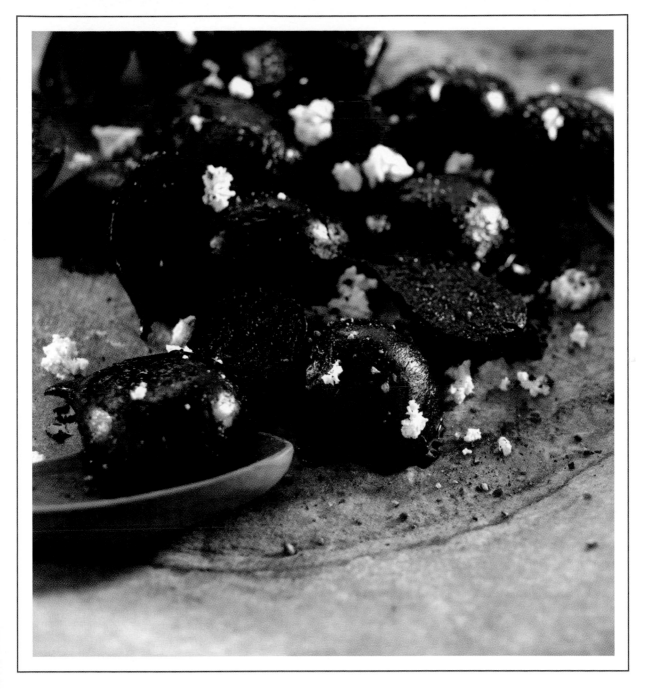

※ PICKLED RED BEETS WITH GOAT CHEESE (page 184) ※

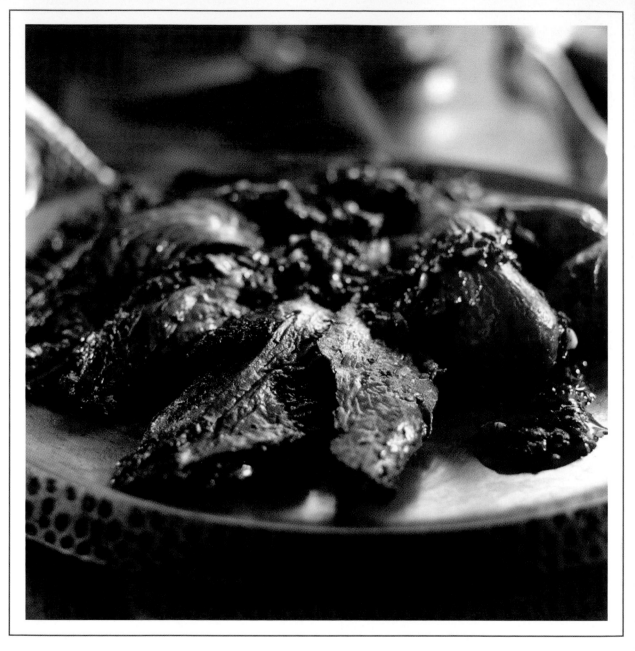

❋ SKIRT STEAK WITH CHIMICHURRI AND ROASTED FINGERLING POTATOES (page 166) ❋

Nelson Mandela's Brown Basmati Rice
with Spinach and Peas

When the former President of South Africa, Nelson Mandela, was on the *Oprah Winfrey Show,* excitement was at a fever pitch. Everyone involved was thrilled that this amazing man was going to be on set. In honor of the visit, I prepared braised, smothered oxtails, which I had heard he liked, served with brown rice biryani. This recipe is reminiscent of the rice I made that day. I am happy to report that President Mandela loved the food. Later Oprah kidded with me about how starstruck I was. "Art, you didn't know whether to bow or curtsy!" she joked. "At least I covered all the bases," I replied with a laugh.

Serves 6

1 teaspoon finely chopped garlic
1 teaspoon finely chopped fresh ginger
1 teaspoon salt
3 tablespoons olive oil
6 whole cloves
2 whole cardamom pods
1 large cinnamon stick
½ teaspoon cumin seeds
½ teaspoon black cumin seeds
½ cup chopped onion
4 whole dried red chilies
2 cups brown basmati rice
1½ cups fresh or defrosted frozen peas
1 cup thawed, drained, and chopped frozen spinach

METHOD Mash the garlic, ginger, and salt into a paste. Scrape into a small bowl.

Heat the oil in a heavy-bottomed medium saucepan over medium heat. Add the cloves, cardamom, cinnamon, cumin, and black cumin and stir until fragrant, about 1½ minutes. Add the onion and cook, stirring occasionally, until translucent, about 3 minutes. Stir in the garlic-ginger paste and the chilies and cook for 1 minute.

Add the rice to the pan and stir to coat it with the aromatics. Add 4 cups of water to the pan and bring to a simmer over high heat. Reduce the heat to low and cover, leaving the lid slightly ajar. Cook for about 25 minutes or until the rice is about three-quarters cooked and most of the liquid had been absorbed.

Add the peas and spinach but do not stir. Cover and continue to cook over low heat for 10 to 15 minutes or until the rice is just cooked and the peas and spinach are warm.

Remove from the heat and let stand for 5 to 10 minutes.

ASSEMBLY Fluff with a fork and serve hot.

Per serving: 331 calories • 10 g fat • 2 g sat fat • 0 mg chol • 444 mg sodium • 57 g carb • 5 g sugar • 7 g fiber • 9 g protein • 61 mg calcium

Sweet Potato Salad with Cumin and Cilantro

~~~~~~

I make this sweet potato salad to serve with the Barbecue Chicken Thighs on page 150, but it stands alone as a terrific side dish that is just as good in the fall as in the summer. Of course, if you like sweet potatoes as much as I do, you'll probably make this all year long.

Serves 6

4 cups medium-diced sweet potato
½ cup nonfat Greek yogurt
½ cup chopped cilantro
2 tablespoons fresh lime juice
1 tablespoon fresh lemon juice
1 teaspoon ground cumin
½ cup minced red onion
2 celery stalks, peeled and thinly sliced
1 jalapeno pepper, seeded and minced
Salt

METHOD Place the sweet potatoes in a large saucepan and cover with water. Bring to a boil and immediately reduce to a simmer. Cook the potatoes for 15 to 20 minutes or until fork tender. Drain the potatoes, place in a large mixing bowl, and cool to room temperature.

In a small mixing bowl, combine the yogurt, cilantro, lime juice, lemon juice, and cumin. Add the yogurt mixture to the sweet potatoes, then add the red onion, celery, and jalapeno pepper. Toss until combined. Cover and refrigerate for 1 hour. Season with salt.

ASSEMBLY Place the sweet potato salad in a serving bowl and enjoy.

Per serving: 98 calories • 0 g fat • 0 g sat fat • 0 mg chol • 76 mg sodium • 21 g carb • 6 g sugar • 3 g fiber • 3 g protein • 53 mg calcium

Roasted Acorn Squash and Honey

~~~~~~

Few side dishes are better on a cool fall evening than roasted acorn squash sweetened with just a little honey and made even mellower with nutmeg and fresh sage leaves. When I catch a whiff of it coming from the oven, I feel warm and comforted, and you will, too.

Serves 4

2 acorn squash (about 1 pound each)
2 tablespoons extra-virgin olive oil
¼ teaspoon grated fresh nutmeg
2 tablespoons honey
8 sage leaves, chopped
Salt and freshly ground black pepper

METHOD Preheat the oven to 350°F.

Split the squash in half and scrape out the seeds with a spoon. Cut the squash halves into quarters and place in a mixing bowl, leaving the skin on the squash sections. Toss the squash with the olive oil, nutmeg, honey, and sage leaves. Lay the squash pieces, cut sides down, on a baking sheet. Bake for 30 to 40 minutes or until the squash flesh begins to turn golden brown and is tender. Season the squash with salt and pepper.

ASSEMBLY Arrange the squash on a serving platter.

Per serving: 108 calories • 5 g fat • 1 g sat fat • 0 mg chol • 4 mg sodium • 18 g carb • 8 g sugar • 2 g fiber • 1 g protein • 39 mg calcium

Green Beans and Tomatoes

~~~~~~

Green beans are easy to find fresh much of the year, but of course they are best in the warm months when grape tomatoes are also sweet as can be. I love tossing them with a little extra-virgin olive oil, lemon juice, and fresh herbs.

Serves 4

8 ounces fresh green beans, trimmed
1½ cups grape tomatoes, cut in half
4 teaspoons extra-virgin olive oil
1 tablespoon fresh lemon juice
1 tablespoon chopped fresh tarragon
Salt and freshly ground black pepper
Grated zest of ½ lemon

METHOD Bring a pot of salted water to a boil. Add the green beans to the pot and cook for 3 to 4 minutes or until cooked al dente (you want some crunch to the beans). Drain and then shock the beans in a bowl of ice water.

Place the beans in a mixing bowl with the tomatoes, olive oil, lemon juice, and tarragon. Toss to combine, then season with salt and pepper.

ASSEMBLY Place the beans on a serving platter and sprinkle with the lemon zest.

Per serving: 70 calories • 5 g fat • 1 g sat fat • 0 mg chol • 6 mg sodium • 7 g carb • 2 g sugar • 3 g fiber • 2 g protein • 31 mg calcium

Pickled Red Beets with Goat Cheese

~~~~~~~~~~~~~~~~~~~~~~~~~~~~~~~~

We serve these beets at Art and Soul, my Washington, D.C., restaurant, and the power brokers love 'em! So does everyone else. Once the beets are baked, their skins just slip off, leaving the sweet, earthy beets for you to enjoy. Beware: when you work with beets, it is normal for your hands to turn red.

Serves 4

16 baby beets
2 tablespoons red wine vinegar
1 teaspoon honey
2 ounces goat cheese (about 4 tablespoons)

METHOD Preheat the oven to 425°F.

Trim the stems from the beets, but leave the skin intact. Wrap the beets in aluminum foil and place on a baking sheet. Bake for 30 minutes or until tender. Let the beets cool to room temperature.

Once the beets are cooked, the skins will come off easily when rubbed with a paper towel. Cut the beets in half and place in a small mixing bowl. Toss with the vinegar and honey. Refrigerate for 1 hour or until chilled.

ASSEMBLY Place the beets in a serving bowl and sprinkle with the goat cheese.

Per serving: 188 calories • 4 g fat • 2 g sat fat • 7 mg chol • 309 mg sodium • 33 g carb • 24 g sugar • 9 g fiber • 8 g protein • 73 mg calcium

$\mathcal{C}$annellini Beans and Roasted Fennel

~~~~~~

It's a good idea to keep canned beans on hand for easy cooking. I used to soak dried beans for hours to hydrate them and then cook them slowly to soften them, but these days I am more apt to rely on canned when cooking at home. I love the way these small white beans taste paired with roasted fennel and seasoned with just a little balsamic vinegar.

Serves 8

2 fennel bulbs, cut into eighths
2 tablespoons extra-virgin olive oil
Salt and freshly ground black pepper
1 tablespoon chopped fennel fronds (the top fernlike part of the
    fennel bulb)
2 15-ounce cans of cannellini beans, rinsed and drained
2 teaspoons balsamic vinegar

METHOD Preheat the oven to 400°F.

Toss the fennel pieces with 1 tablespoon olive oil, then season with salt and pepper. Place the fennel in an ovenproof pan and roast for 20 to 30 minutes or until the fennel is light golden brown and tender. Remove from the oven. Toss the fennel with the fennel fronds.

Heat the beans in a saucepan and stir in the balsamic vinegar and remaining 1 tablespoon olive oil. Season with salt and pepper.

ASSEMBLY Spoon the beans into a serving bowl and top with the roasted fennel.

Per serving: 139 calories • 4 g fat • 1 g sat fat • 0 mg chol • 309 mg sodium • 21 g carb • 2 g sugar • 7 g fiber • 7 g protein • 79 mg calcium

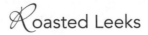oasted Leeks

If you haven't tried roasted leeks, you're in for a treat. They are tender and sweet and taste great alongside just about anything from fish to chicken. Take care to rinse them well, as they can be a little gritty. If I have leftover roasted leeks, I like to fold them into scrambled eggs or add them to salads or even chili.

Serves 4

4 leeks
2 tablespoons extra-virgin olive oil
Salt and freshly ground black pepper
2 sprigs lemon thyme
1 lemon, halved

METHOD Preheat the oven to 375°F.

Trim the root end of the leeks and cut off the top end, the dark green leaves where the outer layer becomes more fibrous. Cut the leeks in half lengthwise and carefully rinse under cold running water. Cut into 4-inch-long pieces.

Place the leeks on a nonstick baking sheet, cut sides up. Either drizzle or brush the leeks with the olive oil and season with salt and pepper. Bake in the oven for 20 to 25 minutes or until the outside of the leeks begins to crisp and turn golden brown, but the inside is still moist. Be careful to check the leeks during the cooking process as the smaller pieces can burn in a matter of a few minutes.

Remove from the oven and cool to room temperature.

ASSEMBLY Arrange the leeks on a serving platter. Pick the leaves from the lemon thyme and sprinkle over the leeks. Squeeze the lemon halves over the leeks and serve.

Per serving: 117 calories • 7 g fat • 1 g sat fat • 0 mg chol • 18 mg sodium • 14 g carb • 3 g sugar • 2 g fiber • 2 g protein • 61 mg calcium

Spinach Custard

Want to get your kids to eat more spinach? Try this. Creamy, cheesy, and soft—they'll love it. It's also fancy enough to serve with a roast chicken, grilled steak, or lamb chops at a dinner party, and yet one of my favorite ways to enjoy the custard is as a light lunch.

Serves 6

2 teaspoons extra-virgin olive oil
½ cup chopped yellow onion
2 10-ounce packages frozen chopped spinach, thawed
2 large eggs, lightly beaten
2 large egg whites, lightly beaten
1 cup nonfat sour cream
3 tablespoons grated Parmesan cheese
1 tablespoon whole wheat pastry flour
¼ teaspoon ground paprika
Salt

METHOD Preheat the oven to 350°F.

Heat a large nonstick sauté pan over medium-high heat. Add the olive oil and onion and cook for 3 to 4 minutes or until translucent.

Drain and squeeze any excess liquid from the spinach. Place the spinach in a large mixing bowl. Add the cooked onions, eggs, egg whites, sour cream, Parmesan cheese, flour, and paprika to the spinach. Mix until fully combined. Season with salt.

Spray a 9-inch pie dish with cooking spray and spoon the spinach mixture into the dish. Bake for 45 minutes or until set. Remove from the oven and let stand for 10 minutes before serving.

ASSEMBLY Cut the custard into 6 slices and serve warm.

Per serving: 121 calories • 4 g fat • 1 g sat fat • 78 mg chol • 209 mg sodium • 13 g carb,1 g sugar • 3 g fiber • 9 g protein • 214 mg calcium

Sugar Snap Peas with Lemon

When the sugar snaps are in the farmer's markets, buy them often. You'll never regret it because they are super easy to cook and everyone loves their sweet crunch. I suggest buying more than you need for the recipe because raw sugar snaps are great for snacking.

Serves 4

8 ounces sugar snap peas
2 tablespoons extra-virgin olive oil
1 tablespoon fresh lemon juice
1 tablespoon chopped fresh mint
Salt and freshly ground black pepper

METHOD Remove the strings from the back of the sugar snap peas. Thinly slice the pea pods on the bias and place in a mixing bowl. Add the olive oil, lemon juice, and mint to the bowl. Toss together until fully incorporated. Season with salt and pepper and let marinate in the refrigerator for 30 minutes before serving.

ASSEMBLY Place the sugar snap peas in a serving bowl. This is best served chilled or at room temperature.

Per serving: 85 calories • 7 g fat • 1g sat fat • 0 mg chol • 2 mg sodium • 5 g carb • 2 g sugar • 2 g fiber • 2 g protein • 26 mg calcium

Slow-Roasted Tomatoes

~~~~~~

I give instructions for roasting cherry tomatoes here, but if you have plum tomatoes or medium-size heirloom or other garden tomatoes, you can roast them, too. Cooked slowly for two hours or so, tomatoes end up being so sweet, so succulent, and so magnificent, you'll want to make these again and again. While this method is best with really good summer tomatoes, it is a good way to treat not-so-good tomatoes because it coaxes out their natural sweetness.

Serves 4

24 cherry tomatoes
6 cloves garlic, smashed
2 tablespoons fresh lemon juice
2 tablespoons extra-virgin olive oil
2 sprigs fresh thyme
2 tablespoons chopped fresh basil

METHOD Preheat the oven to 250°F.

Score the tops of the tomatoes with a knife. Place the tomatoes, garlic cloves, lemon juice, olive oil, and thyme in a small ovenproof pan (you do not want lots of extra room in the pan). Cover with aluminum foil. Slowly roast the tomatoes for 2 hours or until the skins are pulling away from the tomatoes. Discard the thyme sprigs and tomato skins.

ASSEMBLY Place the roasted tomatoes and any juices left in the baking pan on a serving platter and top with the chopped basil.

Per serving: 87 calories • 7 g fat • 1 g sat fat • 0 mg chol • 6 mg sodium • 6 g carb • 3 g sugar • 1 g fiber • 1 g protein • 21 mg calcium

Field Pea and Hominy Succotash

You might need to have spent time in the South to know what field peas are, but once you taste them, you will fall in love. There is not one kind of field peas but several, including black-eyed peas, butter beans, butter peas, lady peas (also called pink peas), and zipper peas (also called white crowders). They all come in slender pods that "zip" open to expose small, perfect peas. If you must, substitute frozen or fresh green peas, often called English peas. This is a great succotash that will make the simplest meal a little special. We serve this at Southern Art, and the Atlanta residents who frequent the restaurant are pleased as punch when they see it on the menu. I suspect it's the field peas that make them happy.

Serves 4

4 ounces dried hominy corn, soaked overnight in water
Salt and freshly ground black pepper
1 cup fresh field peas (I like lady peas)
2 tablespoons extra-virgin olive oil
1 clove garlic, minced
4 green onions, trimmed and chopped
1 large tomato, diced
1 tablespoon fresh lemon juice

METHOD Drain the hominy corn, place in a saucepan, and cover with enough water to reach a depth of 2 inches above the hominy. Bring to a simmer over low heat, season with salt, and simmer, stirring occasionally, for 3 to 3½ hours or until the hominy begins to pop open. You may need to add additional water. Drain the hominy.

Sort and wash the peas and place in a medium saucepan. Add 1 cup cold water and bring to a simmer. Cook the peas for 20 to 30 minutes or until tender. Drain the peas.

Place the olive oil in a large sauté pan over medium heat. Add the garlic and cook for 1 minute or until fragrant. Add the cooked hominy and cooked field peas to the pan and cook for 2 minutes to reheat the hominy and peas. Add the green onions and tomato to the pan and cook for 2 more minutes. Stir in the lemon juice and season to taste with salt and pepper.

ASSEMBLY Place the succotash in a serving bowl and serve while hot.

Per serving: 314 calories • 8 g fat • 1 g sat fat • 0 mg chol • 12 mg sodium • 51 g carb • 5 g sugar • 7 g fiber • 13 g protein • 64 mg calcium

Be Careful Around Carbs

To maintain a healthy weight, eat those carbohydrates that are good for you. It's easy if you remember that you can't go wrong with whole foods: whole grains, whole fruits, and colorful vegetables.

Stay away from processed foods, including white sugar and white flour. Try whole wheat bread and pasta, brown rice, quinoa, millet, and barley. Have an affair with vegetables, especially leafy greens. Most of the time, avoid white potatoes, although not always (let's face it—potatoes are delicious!). Eat sweet potatoes, which are full of good-for-you nutrients. Fill up on legumes such as beans and lentils. And instead of fruit juice, eat the whole fruit so you get that all-important fiber.

Everyone tells you to skip "carbs" when you diet, but considering how many foods are primarily carbohydrates, I say just avoid those that you know aren't good for you: big bowls of pasta, mounds of mashed potatoes, sticky donuts, cream-filled pastries, sugary soft drinks, and salty chips. You know what to cut out of your diet! ❋

Fava Bean, Radish, and Corn Salad

Any side dish or salad that includes corn is pretty, but fava beans and striking-looking breakfast radishes—with their elongated shape, rosy red color, and creamy-looking root ends—make this dish more appealing and appetizing than most. Like most chefs, I love favas, but if you can't find them or think they are too much trouble, replace them with lima beans.

Serves 4

1½ cups shucked fava beans
2 tablespoons extra-virgin olive oil
1 shallot, minced
1½ cups corn kernels
8 breakfast radishes, sliced on the bias
2 tablespoons chopped chives
1 tablespoon chopped fresh basil
1 tablespoon fresh lemon juice
Salt and freshly ground black pepper

METHOD Cook the fava beans in a pot of simmering salted water for 2 to 3 minutes or until cooked al dente. Drain in a colander and shock immediately in a bowl of ice water to stop the cooking. Drain and place in a medium mixing bowl.

Place 1 tablespoon of the olive oil in a preheated sauté pan. Add the shallots and cook over medium heat for 1 minute or until the shallots are translucent. Add the corn to the pan and cook for 3 minutes or until the corn is just cooked. Remove from the heat and cool to room temperature.

Add the corn, radishes, chives, basil, lemon juice, and remaining olive oil to the bowl with the fava beans. Mix until thoroughly combined, then season to taste with salt and pepper.

ASSEMBLY Equally divide the salad between four bowls and enjoy. The salad can be served at room temperature or chilled.

Per serving: 159 calories • 8 g fat • 1 g sat fat • 0 mg chol • 53 mg sodium • 21 g carb • 2 g sugar • 2 g fiber • 6 g protein • 25 mg calcium

Grilled Radicchio

~~~~~~

Yes. Grilled radicchio! So easy and so transforming that even if you don't like radicchio, you'll become a convert. The extra-virgin olive oil and simple honey-and-balsamic dressing are all that is needed to make this side dish something special. Grilling veggies is one of the best ways to savor them, and this is no exception.

Serves 8

2 tablespoons balsamic vinegar
1 tablespoon honey
2 heads radicchio, cut in half
1 tablespoon extra-virgin olive oil
Salt and freshly ground black pepper
2 tablespoons chopped fresh basil

METHOD Preheat a grill to moderate heat.

In a small mixing bowl, combine the balsamic vinegar and honey.

Soak the radicchio in cold water for 30 minutes. Drain and pat dry on paper towels. Coat the radicchio with the olive oil and place on the grill for 5 to 7 minutes on each side, or until cooked through. Baste the radicchio with the vinegar-honey mixture and cook for an additional minute on each side.

Remove from the grill and season with salt and pepper.

ASSEMBLY Place the radicchio on a serving plate and top with the chopped basil.

Per serving: 27 calories • 2 g fat • 0 g sat fat • 0 mg chol • 1 mg sodium • 3 g carb • 3 g sugar • 0 g fiber • 0 g protein • 3 mg calcium

Braised Collard Greens with Smoked Turkey

~~~~~~

I like to call these Glory Greens because they are nothing short of glorious! We have them on the menu at TABLE Fifty-Two, my Chicago restaurant, and even born-and-bred northerners clean their plates. Who would have thought of eating collard greens in the Windy City? Well, I would, for one! And you will want to eat these wherever you live, too.

Serves 8

1 teaspoon extra-virgin olive oil
1 small yellow onion, chopped
½ teaspoon chili flakes
½ cup red wine vinegar
½ cup apple cider vinegar
2 tablespoons stevia
2 pounds collard greens (or turnip or mustard greens), chopped
    and rinsed
4 ounces skinless, shredded smoked turkey breast
Sea salt

METHOD Preheat a large sauté pan over medium heat. Add the olive oil and onions, and cook for 5 to 7 minutes or until the onions are translucent. Add the chili flakes, red wine and apple cider vinegars, stevia, chopped greens, and turkey meat. Cover and slowly cook over low heat for 60 to 90 minutes or until the greens are very tender. Sprinkle with a little sea salt.

ASSEMBLY Place the hot greens in a serving bowl. These are best enjoyed hot.

Per serving: 78 calories • 3 g fat • 0 g sat fat • 7 mg chol • 148 sodium • 10 g carb • 1 g sugar • 4 g fiber • 5 g protein • 168 mg calcium

Roasted Cauliflower with Pepperoncini

As I have said over and over on these pages, roasting vegetables is one of the best ways to render them sweet, tender, and tempting. Please discover roasted cauliflower if you have not already done so. It's amazing! When we serve this at TABLE Fifty-Two in Chicago, we finish it with white cheddar cheese powder, which makes it especially luscious. I don't do so in this recipe because, frankly, I don't have to gild the lily to enjoy every bite of this dish.

Serves 4

1 head cauliflower, cut into 2-inch florets
16 pepperoncini peppers, sliced
3 tablespoons extra-virgin olive oil
Salt and freshly ground black pepper

METHOD Preheat the oven to 425°F.

Place the cauliflower florets on a parchment-lined baking sheet and bake for 35 minutes or until the cauliflower begins to turn golden brown on the edges. Remove from the oven and place in a medium mixing bowl. Add the pepperoncini and olive oil, season with salt and pepper, and toss until fully mixed.

ASSEMBLY Place the cauliflower mixture in a serving bowl and serve as a side dish or snack. This is great at room temperature or hot.

Per serving: 163 calories • 11 g fat • 2 g sat fat • 0 mg chol • 731 mg sodium • 15 g carb • 5 g sugar • 5 g fiber • 4 g protein • 46 mg calcium

Party Day Foods: Treats Big and Small

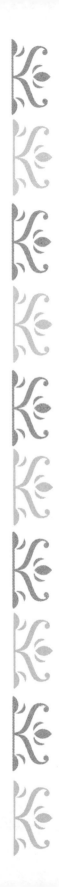

Even the most committed athlete and healthy eater needs a treat now and again, so I came up with a system that works for me. I call it "party day." Once a week, I allow myself a few indulgences. Although I don't necessarily have a party, my taste buds get to dance around in my mouth, laughing and singing with joy.

Not everyone savors food the way I do. Some folks think of it merely as fuel, as a way to keep their bodies going from one event to the next, but most of us have strong feelings about the tastes and textures of the countless foods and dishes out there and don't want to miss out. Many people trying to lose weight believe they will never again be able to indulge in pizza, mac and cheese, or a summertime angel food cake. Boo hoo. Not true! The glory of a balanced, sensible, healthy diet is that you can eat anything you want—just not *anytime* you want. Save it for your party day!

I didn't reach a weight of more than three hundred pounds, complete with achy knees and high blood glucose levels, because I love poached chicken and steamed vegetables. I got there from overeating, from never putting on the brakes. With the help of my trainer Az and common sense, I learned to appreciate simple meals that allowed me to drop the pounds and pick up the activity. I feel great at this "fighting weight." There's not a piece of chocolate cake or a sweet, tropical cocktail that tastes as good as I feel now, but that doesn't mean I don't love biting into perfectly fried chicken, forking up tender short ribs and mashed potatoes, or indulging in poached pears with extravagant mascarpone cheese. Just not every day. All week I may look forward to my party day, but curiously I don't count the minutes. And when I allow myself a few treats, I eat less than I used to. And—really, this is true—I enjoy them more!

I've included twenty recipes in this chapter for dishes that are drop-dead delicious. I organized them so that breakfast foods are first, followed by lunch and dinner offerings, and finally luscious, irresistible desserts. I include simple grilled watermelon but also have recipes for peach cobbler, chocolate bark, and baked apples.

Whole Wheat Biscuits with Crushed Strawberries and Honey ❈ 200

Sweet Potato Waffles with Lemon Ricotta ❈ 202

Chicken and Root Vegetable Pot Pie ❈ 204

Zucchini Lasagna ❈ 206

Buttermilk Fried Chicken ❈ 208

Whole Wheat Margherita Pizza ❈ 211

Tomato Soup and Grilled Cheese ❈ 213

Three-Cheese Macaroni ❈ 215

Arepas ❈ 217

Art Smith's Healthy Comfort

$\mathcal{B}$raised Beef Short Ribs with Carrots and Garlic-Mashed Potatoes ❋ 218

$\mathcal{C}$lam Chowder with Garlic Toasts ❋ 220

$\mathcal{O}$range–Poppy Seed Angel Food Cupcakes ❋ 222

$\mathcal{P}$each Cobbler ❋ 224

$\mathcal{L}$emon-Yogurt Panna Cotta with Blueberries ❋ 226

$\mathcal{P}$oached Pears with Lemon Mascarpone ❋ 228

$\mathcal{B}$aked Apples with Cinnamon-Oatmeal Streusel ❋ 229

$\mathcal{S}$trawberry Soup with Greek Frozen Yogurt ❋ 230

$\mathcal{G}$rilled Watermelon ❋ 232

$\mathcal{D}$ark Chocolate, Pumpkin Seed, and Sea Salt Bark ❋ 234

$\mathcal{H}$ibiscus-Mint Granita ❋ 235

Whole Wheat Biscuits with Crushed Strawberries and Honey

~~~~~~

Being a southerner through and through, I can't write a book that does not include biscuits. These are made with whole wheat pastry flour and bread flour in the perfect proportion to ensure that these buttermilk biscuits are as light as can be. I love them for breakfast every now and again. I don't eat them often, though, and am a far healthier man today than I was several years ago. But that doesn't mean we have given up biscuits! Or that we aren't "thick as grits" when it comes to our roots.

Serves 10

For the biscuits:
2½ cups whole wheat pastry flour
½ cup bread flour
2½ teaspoons baking powder
½ teaspoon baking soda
¾ teaspoon kosher salt
1 cup cream cheese, cubed
¼ cup unsalted butter, cubed and chilled
¾ to 1 cup buttermilk, plus more for brushing
2 tablespoons rolled oats

For the strawberries:
2 cups strawberries, stemmed and quartered
2 tablespoons honey
1 tablespoon fresh lemon juice
2 tablespoons chopped fresh mint

METHOD To prepare the biscuits: Preheat the oven to 400°F. Line a baking sheet with parchment paper.

In a large mixing bowl, combine the whole wheat and bread flours, baking powder, baking soda, and salt. Cut the cream cheese and butter into the flour mixture using two forks or your hands. Work until the cream cheese and butter are fully incorporated and the mixture resembles coarse crumbs. Add ¾ cup buttermilk and mix with a spoon until the mixture is moistened (add additional buttermilk if needed).

Turn the dough onto a floured surface and knead 3 or 4 times until the dough comes together. Do not overwork. Pat the dough until it is about 1¼ inch thick. Cut the dough into 10 biscuits with a 1½-inch round cutter.

Transfer the biscuits to the parchment-lined baking sheet. Brush the tops of the biscuits with buttermilk and sprinkle with the rolled oats. Bake for 20 minutes or until golden brown. Remove from the oven and serve warm. You can store leftover biscuits in an airtight container.

To prepare the strawberries: In a medium mixing bowl, combine the strawberries, honey, lemon, and mint. Crush the strawberries with a fork until all the ingredients have come together.

ASSEMBLY Slice the biscuits in half and spoon the strawberry mixture over the biscuits.

Per serving: 268 calories • 13 g fat • 8 g sat fat • 39 mg chol • 446 mg sodium • 32 g carb • 7 g sugar • 3 g fiber • 6 g protein • 100 mg calcium

Sweet Potato Waffles with Lemon Ricotta

Waffles for breakfast. Must be the weekend! These are made with whole wheat pastry flour and raw sugar, but instead of detracting from the goodness, as some people might suspect, the ingredients result in the best waffles to come out of a waffle iron in decades. The lemony ricotta is a superb topping.

Serves 6

For the waffles:
2 cups whole wheat pastry flour
2 tablespoons raw sugar
1 tablespoon baking powder
½ teaspoon kosher salt
½ teaspoon ground cinnamon
1 cup buttermilk
½ cup nonfat plain Greek yogurt
½ cup mashed baked sweet potatoes
1 tablespoon canola oil
1 teaspoon pure vanilla extract
3 large eggs, separated

For the lemon ricotta:
8 tablespoons ricotta cheese
1 tablespoon honey
Grated zest of 1 lemon

For the garnish:
Maple syrup (optional)

METHOD To prepare the waffles: Preheat a waffle iron.

In a large mixing bowl, combine the flour, sugar, baking powder, salt, and cinnamon and whisk until fully incorporated.

In a medium mixing bowl, combine the buttermilk, yogurt, sweet potato, oil, vanilla extract, and egg yolks. Whisk until fully incorporated.

In a medium mixing bowl, beat the egg whites at high speed for about 2 minutes or until stiff peaks form. Set aside.

Pour the milk mixture over the flour mixture and whisk until well combined; the batter should be nearly smooth. Fold in the stiff egg whites. The batter is now ready for the waffle iron.

Pour the batter into the waffle iron to make a waffle that is about 7 inches across. Cook until golden brown. Repeat this process with the remaining batter.

To prepare the lemon ricotta: In a small mixing bowl, combine the ricotta, honey, and lemon zest.

ASSEMBLY Place two waffles on each plate and top with a spoonful of the lemon ricotta. Drizzle with maple syrup if desired.

Per serving: 277 calories • 7 g fat • 2 g sat fat • 116 mg chol • 551 mg sodium • 41 g carb • 11 g sugar • 4 g fiber • 13 g protein • 208 mg calcium

Chicken and Root Vegetable Pot Pie

If chicken pot pie isn't comfort food, I don't know what is. It's warm, mild, and full of friendly, familiar flavors that hit the spot when the weather is stormy or you're feeling a little low. The store-bought puff pastry makes this easy to prepare.

Serves 4

3 cups low-sodium chicken stock
1 cup diced Yukon Gold potatoes
1 cup diced sweet potatoes
1 cup diced celery root
1 cup diced parsnip
1 large white onion, diced
1 pound boneless, skinless chicken breasts, diced
⅔ cup all-purpose flour
1½ cups whole milk
1 cup fresh or frozen peas
¼ cup chopped flat-leaf parsley
2 tablespoons chopped cilantro
1 teaspoon hot sauce
Salt and freshly ground black pepper
1 sheet frozen puff pastry dough, thawed

METHOD Preheat the oven to 400°F.

Place the chicken stock in a large soup pot. Bring to a boil and add the Yukon Gold and sweet potatoes, celery root, parsnip, and onion. Cover and reduce the heat to medium-low, then simmer for 5 minutes. Add the chicken and simmer for 10 minutes longer or until the chicken is just cooked. Remove the chicken and vegetables from the stock with a slotted spoon and reserve.

Place the flour in a mixing bowl and gradually add the milk, whisking it into the flour until well blended. Add this mixture to the stock and bring to a simmer for 5 minutes or until thickened. Add peas, parsley, cilantro, hot sauce, and the reserved chicken and vegetables to the stock and season with salt and pepper.

Place four 16-ounce ramekins on a baking sheet. Fill the ramekins with the chicken and vegetable mixture.

~~~~~~

Cut the puff pastry into 4 pieces and lay each one over a ramekin. Gently press the dough over the edges of the ramekins.

Bake for 20 to 25 minutes or until the puff pastry is golden brown and the filling is bubbly.

ASSEMBLY Place the hot ramekins on serving plates and enjoy.

Per serving: 467 calories • 10 g fat • 4 g sat fat • 72 mg chol • 306 mg sodium • 58 g carb • 11 g sugar • 8 g fiber • 37 g protein • 184 mg calcium

Zucchini Lasagna

~~~~~~

Lasagna made with zucchini is just as satisfying as lasagna made with meat and a whole lot better for you. We put this on the menu at Joanne Trattoria, the New York restaurant opened by Joseph and Cynthia Germanotta in which I have an interest. Their famous daughter is Lady Gaga, who enjoys this rich, cheesy casserole as a special treat.

Serves 8

For the roux:
1 stick unsalted butter
1 cup all-purpose flour

For the cheese sauce:
1 quart whole milk
1 pound fontina cheese, grated
Salt

For the lasagna:
3 large zucchini
3 large yellow squash
3 cups ricotta cheese
3 large eggs, beaten
¼ cup chopped flat-leaf parsley
1 cup grated Parmesan cheese
2 teaspoons onion powder
1 teaspoon garlic powder
Salt and freshly ground black pepper
8 ounces dried lasagna pasta sheets (9 sheets), cooked

For the garnish:
½ cup chopped fresh basil

METHOD To prepare the roux: In a small saucepan, melt the butter over medium heat. Whisk in the flour while cooking over medium heat for 8 to 10 minutes, or until it comes together. Set aside and let cool.

To prepare the cheese sauce: In a large saucepan, bring the milk to a simmer and slowly add the roux while whisking. Cook for 20 to 25 minutes over medium-low heat, whisking continually. Add the grated cheese, about ½ pound at a time. Continue to whisk until all the cheese is added. Taste for desired salt.

To prepare the lasagna: Preheat the oven to 350°F.

Slice the zucchini and yellow squash lengthwise into ¼-inch-thick pieces.

In a medium mixing bowl, combine the ricotta, eggs, parsley, Parmesan, and onion and garlic powders. Season to taste with salt and pepper.

In a 9- × 13-inch lasagna pan, place 1 cup of the cheese sauce. Lay 3 lasagna sheets over the sauce and spread ½ cup of the ricotta mixture over the lasagna sheets. Next layer with half of the squash and zucchini. Repeat until you have used all the ingredients, ending with 1 cup of the cheese sauce spread over the assembled lasagna. You will have still more cheese sauce to serve alongside the lasagna.

Bake for 40 to 50 minutes or until the lasagna is bubbling and golden brown. Remove from the oven and let sit for 20 minutes before cutting into 8 pieces.

ASSEMBLY Warm the cheese sauce just prior to serving, and spoon some on each plate. Place a piece of the lasagna over the sauce and sprinkle with the basil.

Per serving: 789 calories • 46 g fat • 28 g sat fat • 227 mg chol • 819 mg sodium • 52 g carb • 12 g sugar • 4 g fiber • 43 g protein • 871 mg calcium

Buttermilk Fried Chicken

~~~~~~

I am well known for my fried chicken—and, in all modesty, for good reason. It's lip-smackin' good! I don't cook it very often anymore, but when I do, folks flock to it. Fried chicken is one of the great comfort foods to come out of the South, along with real barbecue, ham and biscuits, braised greens, and coconut cake. When Oprah invited me on her show to talk about my weight loss and victory over diabetes, I was *not* thinking about southern fried chicken. This changed when I heard that Lady Gaga, my all-time favorite pop star, was backstage. I grabbed Chef Rey Villalobos, the chef at TABLE Fifty-Two, my Chicago restaurant, and we cooked up fried chicken and waffles for her. Minutes after the food was delivered, Lady Gaga came screaming out of her dressing room. "Art Smith, I love you! You're my favorite on *Top Chef Masters*."

Good fried chicken is all about the timing. Dark meat needs about eight minutes to cook, while white meat requires a few more minutes due to its size and configuration. I suggest cooking them separately so you get the timing right. This recipe also works great with King Arthur Gluten-Free Flour.

Serves 10

For the brine:
1 gallon cold water
½ cup kosher salt
1 teaspoon black peppercorns
3 sprigs rosemary
5 sprigs thyme
4 cloves garlic
2 bay leaves

For the chicken:
2 whole chickens, cut into 10 pieces each
1 quart buttermilk

For the egg wash:
6 large eggs
1 tablespoon hot sauce

2 teaspoons salt
2 teaspoons ground black pepper

For the dredge:
2 cups all-purpose flour or gluten-free flour
3 cups self-rising flour (I use White Lily flour, or gluten-free flour)
1 tablespoon garlic powder
1 tablespoon onion powder
1 tablespoon salt
2 tablespoons paprika
½ teaspoon cayenne
2 teaspoons dried thyme

For frying the chicken:
Canola oil

METHOD **To prepare the brine:** In a large soup kettle, dissolve the salt in 2 cups water over medium-high heat. Add the remaining water, stirring to blend in the salt. Add the black peppercorns, rosemary, thyme, garlic cloves, and bay leaves.

To prepare the chicken: Place the chicken pieces in the brine and refrigerate for at least 12 hours.

Remove the chicken from the brine and submerge in the buttermilk. Refrigerate for 4 to 6 hours.

To prepare the egg wash: In a large mixing bowl, whisk together the eggs, hot sauce, salt, and pepper.

Drain the chicken from the buttermilk and put in the bowl with the egg wash. Turn the chicken pieces to coat them with the egg wash.

To prepare the dredge: Mix together the all-purpose and self-rising flours, garlic and onion powders, salt, paprika, cayenne, and thyme. Add more salt if needed.

Remove 2 pieces of chicken at a time from the egg wash, letting the excess liquid drain off. Roll in the seasoned flour. Shake off any excess flour and lay the chicken on a wire rack until ready to fry. (It is crucial that any excess flour is shaken off before frying the chicken.) Repeat with the remaining chicken pieces.

To fry the chicken: Pour canola oil into a large cast iron pan to a depth of 1 inch and heat over medium heat until it registers 325°F on a deep-frying thermometer. Place 4 to 6 pieces of chicken into the oil. Take care to use long tongs to move the chicken and do not crowd the pan.

Turn each piece about every 2 minutes. If the chicken begins to darken, turn the flame on the stove down slightly to adjust the temperature. Cook the chicken until it reaches an internal temperature of 180°F. Be sure to give the oil 5 minutes to reach the proper temperature before dropping in the next batch of chicken.

Place the fried chicken on a plate lined with paper towels to absorb excess oil and keep at room temperature until ready to serve.

ASSEMBLY Place the fried chicken on two large serving platters and serve.

Per serving: 749 calories • 37 g fat • 10 g sat fat • 271 mg chol • 2002 mg sodium • 54 g carb • 5 g sugar • 3 g fiber • 48 g protein • 234 mg calcium

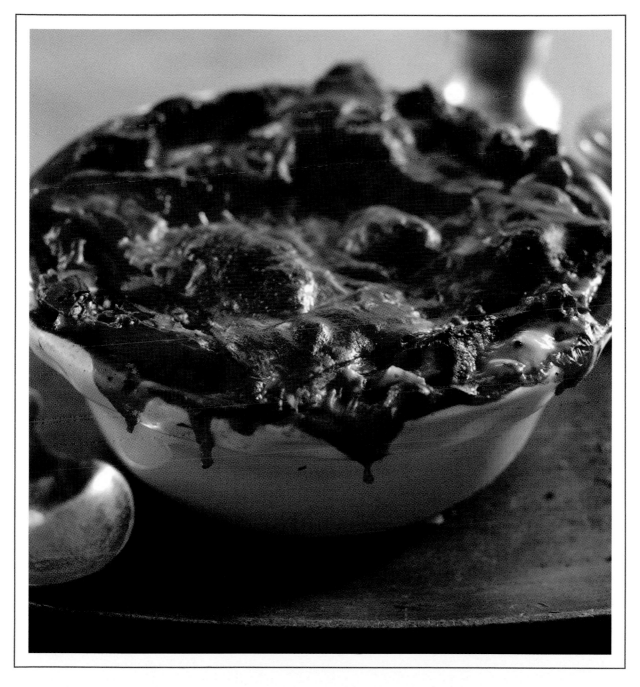

※ CHICKEN AND ROOT VEGETABLE POT PIE (page 204) ※

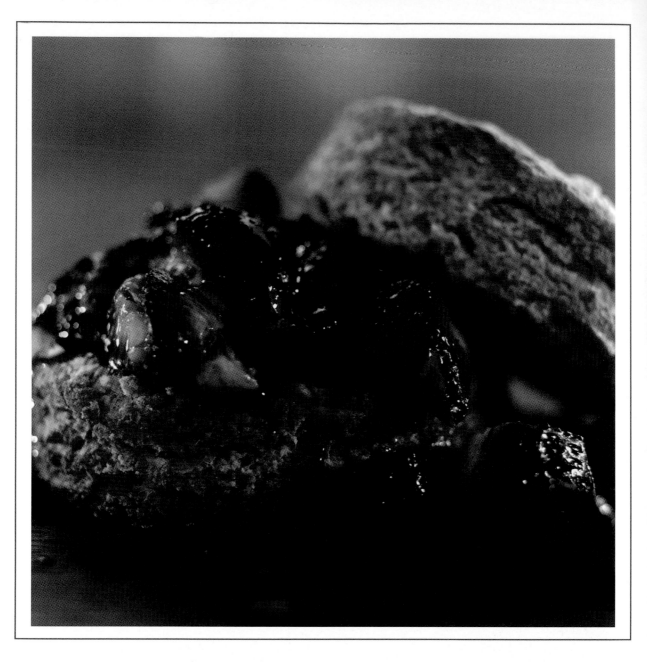

❊ WHOLE WHEAT BISCUITS WITH CRUSHED STRAWBERRIES AND HONEY (page 200) ❊

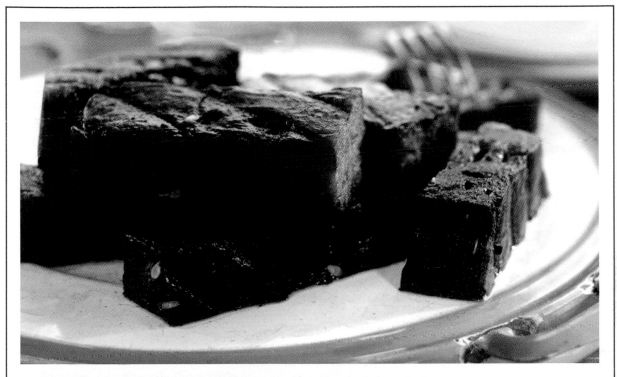

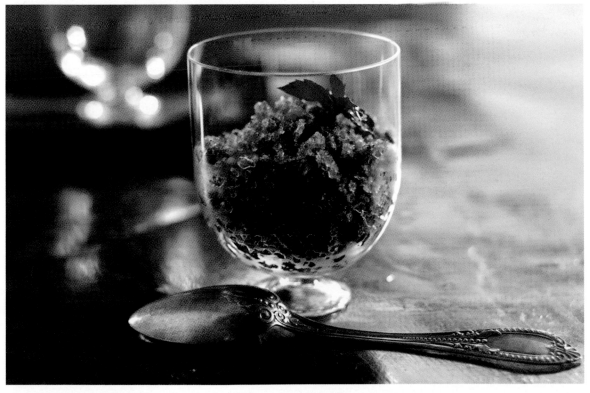

❋ *Top:* GRILLED WATERMELON (page 232) ❋ *Bottom:* HIBISCUS-MINT GRANITA (page 235) ❋

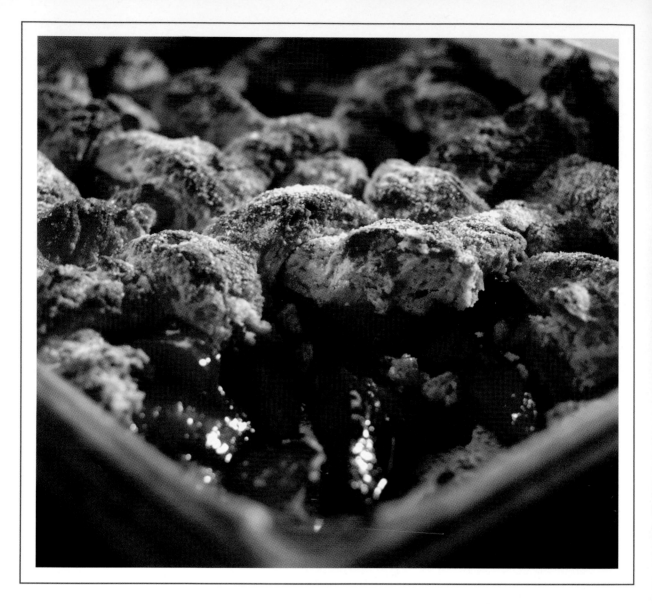

❋ PEACH COBBLER (page 224) ❋

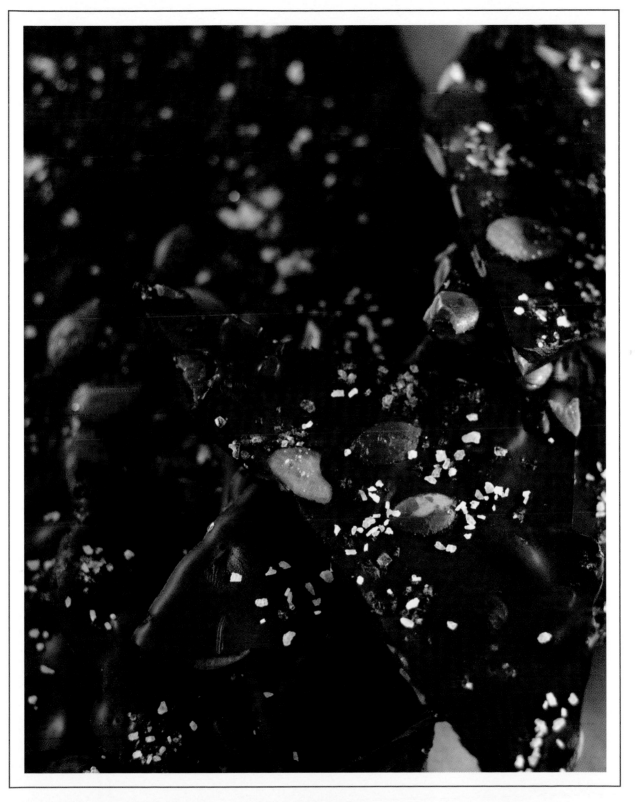

❉ DARK CHOCOLATE, PUMPKIN SEED, AND SEA SALT BARK (page 234) ❉

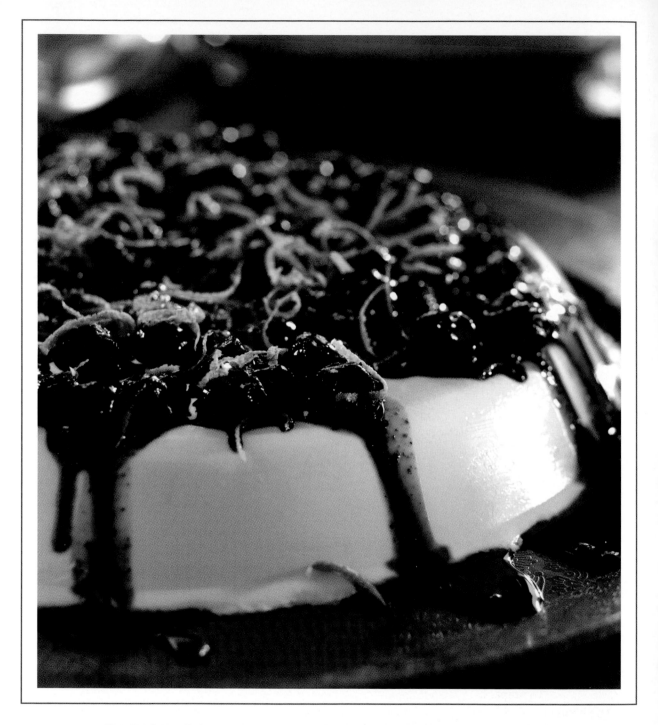

❋ LEMON-YOGURT PANNA COTTA WITH BLUEBERRIES (page 226) ❋

Whole Wheat Margherita Pizza

After I had lost about 85 pounds and gotten my diabetes under control, Mehmet Oz asked me to come on the *Dr. Oz Show* to celebrate my success. I just had to decide what to cook on the air. A few weeks earlier, my friend legal eagle pizzaiolo Kenneth Robling and I came up with the idea for this fabulously healthy pizza. A lot of folks think "healthy pizza" is an oxymoron and the final dish must be boring, but not this one! The perfectly chewy crust is topped with tomatoes, mozzarella, basil and Parmesan cheese, and every bite is an eye-opener. I threw a little pizza party to showcase it and invited Daphne Oz, Dr. Oz's daughter, a committed vegetarian and one of the hosts of *The Chew*. She loved it! Since then, I have also topped it with roasted mushrooms and chopped arugula. You can come up with your own ideas.

Serves 6

For the dough:
1¼ cups warm water at approximately 110°F
1 tablespoon agave nectar
1 package dry active yeast
1½ cups whole wheat white flour
1½ cups unbleached all-purpose flour
1 teaspoon sea salt
1 tablespoon extra-virgin olive oil
Additional flour for kneading

For the assembly:
1 28-ounce can San Marzano tomatoes or other canned tomatoes
1 8-ounce ball buffalo mozzarella, thinly sliced
Sea salt and freshly ground black pepper
1 cup fresh basil leaves, torn into 1-inch pieces
1 2-ounce block Parmesan cheese

METHOD **To prepare the dough:** Pour warm water and agave nectar in the bowl of a food processor fitted with the plastic dough blade. Sprinkle the yeast over the water and allow it to bloom for 10 minutes until bubbly. Add the whole wheat and all-purpose flours, salt, and olive oil, and pulse until the dough comes together into a sticky ball. Remove the dough from the processor. Sprinkle on some additional flour and knead into a soft dough. Place the ball of kneaded dough in a large mixing bowl and cover with a clean kitchen towel. Allow to rise until doubled in bulk, approximately 1 hour. Divide into 3 balls, each of which will make a 10-inch pie.

To assemble the pizzas: Preheat the oven to 550°F.

Drain the tomatoes. Tear the tomatoes into 4 pieces each, discarding any visible seeds.

Put 1 ball of dough on top of a piece of parchment paper and flatten it with your hands. Gently stretch to form a 10-inch circle. If using a pizza stone, preheat the stone for 1 hour at 500°F. If you're not using a stone, you can transform a regular rectangular baking sheet into a great pizza pan by turning it over.

Shape the pizza on the parchment paper and then sprinkle with the tomato pieces and mozzarella slices. Sprinkle with sea salt and pepper. Repeat this process with the remaining dough so you have 3 pizzas.

Place each pizza (and parchment paper) on the hot stone or baking sheet and bake for 2 to 3 minutes just until the dough is firm. Pull the parchment from under the pizza and bake for 15 to 20 minutes longer or until the top is bubbly and the crust is golden brown. Remove from the oven.

ASSEMBLY Sprinkle the torn basil over the hot pizzas, grate Parmesan cheese on top, and serve immediately.

Per serving: 438 calories • 14 g fat • 7 g sat fat • 37 mg chol • 771 mg sodium • 58 g carb • 7 g sugar • 6 g fiber • 18 g protein • 140 mg calcium

Tomato Soup and Grilled Cheese

One of the all-time great combinations for a rainy day, late night munch, or Saturday lunch, tomato soup and grilled cheese sandwiches hit the spot. Making your own tomato soup is nearly as easy as opening a can, and so much better. The cheese sandwiches are buttery and gooey, just like everyone likes them!

Serves 8

For the soup:
3 pounds large tomatoes, cut in half
2 unpeeled medium Vidalia onions, cut in half
2 cups low-sodium chicken stock
2 tablespoons extra-virgin olive oil
Salt and freshly ground black pepper

For the grilled cheese:
16 slices ciabatta bread
½ cup unsalted butter, softened
8 1-ounce slices cheddar cheese
8 1-ounce slices Swiss cheese

METHOD To prepare the soup: Preheat a grill to moderate heat.

Place the tomatoes and onion on the grill, cut side down. Grill them both for 5 to 7 minutes or until the tomatoes are lightly charred and the onion has dark grill marks on it. Turn the onions cut side up and grill for an additional 5 to 7 minutes or until tender. Cool the tomatoes and onion, discarding the peels and seeds. Coarsely chop the onion and place in a food processer fitted with a metal blade. Add the tomatoes, stock, and olive oil. Puree until smooth. Transfer to a saucepan and warm over medium heat. Season with salt and pepper.

To prepare the grilled cheese: Heat a cast-iron skillet or griddle to medium. Liberally butter one side of each piece of bread. Place a slice of cheddar and a slice of Swiss cheese on half the bread slices on the sides that are not buttered. Top with the remaining bread, buttered sides up. Place the sandwich on the skillet or griddle and cook until the bread is golden brown and the cheeses melt together, 3 to 5 minutes on each side. Cut the sandwiches in half diagonally.

ASSEMBLY Ladle the soup into 8 soup bowls and serve with the hot grilled cheese sandwiches.

Per serving: 460 calories • 33 g fat • 19 g sat fat • 85 mg chol • 406 mg sodium • 23 g carb • 10 g sugar • 3 g fiber • 20 g protein • 494 mg calcium

Sugar Ain't So Sweet

Have you ever carried around a five-pound sack of sugar? Of course. Multiply that by more than thirteen and you will arrive at the amount of sugar we Americans consume in a year. Yep. That's right: sixty-six pounds for every man, woman, and child. I got this figure from the U.S. Department of Agriculture, which is considered about as reliable a source as any. Other studies claim that each of us consumes as much as 130 pounds a year. And you know what? Even that number does not surprise me.

So what? We're just talking about refined sugar, empty calories that don't cause much harm, except for dental cavities, right? Sure, sixty-six pounds on average is a lot, but it's no reason for alarm.

Think again. Refined sugar is toxic, as far as I am concerned. Not only does it contribute to obesity (and 120 million Americans are obese, with the number rising annually), but it is an underlying cause of type 2 diabetes, a dangerous disease I must battle. What's more, very reputable scientists believe sugar contributes to heart disease, hypertension, and even some cancers.

What's the upshot? Forget sweeteners as part of your daily diet. Add whole berries and sliced peaches to your morning cereal, learn to drink your coffee and tea unsweetened, abandon soda (regular and sugar-free), and though you can indulge in a piece of cake or bowl of ice cream now and again, don't make it a regular habit. Do what our forebearers did: save sweets for special occasions.

When you get right down to it, this makes all kinds of sense and goes along with the mantra of health-conscious folks: eat foods as close to their whole state as you can, and enjoy their natural, God-given sweetness. Guess what! You won't feel the least bit deprived. ❅

$\mathcal{T}$hree-Cheese Macaroni

When we put this on the menu at TABLE Fifty-Two, our guests went wild. Mac and cheese shows up on any number of restaurant menus across the country, but mine is one of the best. Why? Simple. I love mac and cheese—I find it super comforting and satisfying and have spent hours perfecting it. You won't be disappointed when you indulge on your party day!

Serves 8

For the roux:
1 cup (2 sticks) unsalted butter
1⅓ cups all-purpose flour

For the Mornay cheese sauce:
1 quart whole milk
½ pound fontina cheese, grated
½ pound white cheddar cheese, grated
½ pound yellow cheddar cheese, grated
Salt

For assembly:
1 pound penne noodles, cooked according to package directions
½ pound cheddar cheese, grated

METHOD To prepare the roux: In a small saucepan, melt the butter. Whisk in the flour and cook over medium heat for 8 to 10 minutes or until it has come together. Set aside and let cool.

To prepare the Mornay cheese sauce: In a large saucepan, bring the milk to a simmer and slowly add the roux while whisking. Cook for 20 to 25 minutes over medium-low heat, whisking continuously. Add the grated cheese, ½ pound at a time, continuing to whisk until all the cheese is added. Taste for desired salt.

To assemble the macaroni and cheese: Preheat the oven to 425°F.

Butter an 8- × 9-inch ovenproof baking dish. Add the cooked penne pasta. Pour the Mornay cheese sauce over the pasta and sprinkle it with the remaining grated cheese. Place the baking dish on a baking sheet and bake in the oven for 20 to 25 minutes or until the cheese is golden brown and the sauce is bubbling over the sides of the pan.

Remove from the oven and let sit for 10 minutes before serving.

ASSEMBLY Divide among 8 serving bowls.

Per serving: 1,011 calories • 65 g fat • 39 g sat fat • 196 mg chol • 832 mg sodium • 67 g carb • 8 g sugar • 2 g fiber • 42 g protein • 911 mg calcium

Arepas

~~~~~~

For a special weekend breakfast, my husband, Jesus, makes these arepas. He is from Venezuela, where he learned to make these from his beautiful mother, Hilda. Here I fill them with rich, smooth cream cheese, but we've eaten them filled with meat, butter, or eggs, too.

Serves 8

2½ to 3 cups lukewarm water
1 tablespoon sugar
2 teaspoons kosher salt
2 cups precooked white cornmeal (masarepa cornmeal)
2 teaspoons canola oil
½ cup cream cheese

METHOD Preheat the oven to 350°F.

Place the water, sugar, and salt in a medium mixing bowl and stir until the sugar and salt dissolve. Add the cornmeal to the bowl little by little, mixing with your hands. Stop adding the cornmeal just before the dough has the consistency of a thick pancake batter. Continue to stir vigorously with your hands until the dough starts to pull away from the sides of the bowl and forms a very soft ball. Add additional cornmeal if the dough doesn't firm up, but it should not be as firm as bread dough. When the dough forms a nice moist ball, break off small pieces and work them into 2-inch balls. Gently flatten the small balls of dough until they are about ½ inch thick. (If the dough cracks on the edges, dampen your hands and try again.) Continue with the rest of the dough.

Lightly grease a flat griddle or frying pan with the canola oil and put over medium-high heat. Place the arepa on the preheated griddle and cook for 2 minutes over medium-high heat. Flip the arepas just before they are about to burn, when the bottom is golden brown. Cook for 2 more minutes or until golden brown on the other side. Place the arepas on a baking sheet and bake for 10 minutes or until they puff up.

ASSEMBLY Slice open the arepas, spread with cream cheese, and serve.

Per serving: 210 calories • 6 g fat • 3 g sat fat • 16 mg chol • 530 mg sodium • 34 g carb • 2 g sugar • 1 g fiber • 4 g protein • 16 mg calcium

Braised Beef Short Ribs with Carrots and Garlic-Mashed Potatoes

~~~~~~

For some people, short ribs and mashed potatoes are the ultimate comfort food. Who can argue? Slow-cooked until the meat falls off the bones, the short ribs are rich and flavorful and their gravy mingles gloriously with the garlicky mashed potato. Who can resist?

Serves 4

For the short ribs:
2 tablespoons canola oil
4 beef short ribs
Salt and freshly ground black pepper
1 cup chopped yellow onion
1 cup chopped leeks
4 carrots, peeled and cut into large dice
2 cups chopped tomato
6 garlic cloves, peeled and smashed
2 jalapeno chili peppers, cut in half
1 cup red wine
1 sprig fresh rosemary
2 sprigs fresh thyme
1½ cups chicken broth

For the potatoes:
2 pounds Yukon Gold potatoes, peeled and cut into medium dice
8 garlic cloves
1 cup milk, heated
½ cup butter
Salt and freshly ground black pepper

For the garnish:
2 tablespoons chopped chives

METHOD To prepare the short ribs: Preheat the oven to 275°F.

Heat the oil in a roasting pan over medium-high heat. Season the ribs with salt and pepper. Add the ribs to the pan and sear for 2 minutes on each side or until golden brown. Remove the ribs from the pan and set aside. Add the onion, leeks, and carrots to the pan and cook over medium heat for 7 to 10 minutes or until golden brown. Add the tomatoes, garlic, and jalapeno and cook for 5 minutes, stirring to incorporate. Add the wine, rosemary, thyme, and chicken broth and bring to a simmer. Return the ribs to the pan and cover tightly with aluminum foil.

Braise in the oven for 4 to 6 hours, or until the meat is fork tender. Just prior to serving, remove the ribs from the pan and simmer the braising liquid on the stove top for 10 to 15 minutes or until it has a saucelike consistency.

To prepare the potatoes: Place the potatoes and garlic cloves in a pot and cover with 2 inches of cold, salted water. Bring to a simmer and cook for 20 minutes or until tender. Drain the potatoes and pass through a ricer. Place in the bowl of an electric mixer. Add the milk and butter and whip until smooth. Season with salt and pepper.

ASSEMBLY Spoon some of the potatoes into the center of each serving plate. Top with a short rib and spoon some of the reduced braising liquid around the plate. Sprinkle with the chopped chives.

Per serving: 895 calories • 48 g fat • 23 g sat fat • 145 mg chol • 661 mg sodium • 72 g carb • 15 g sugar • 9 g fiber • 36 g protein • 202 mg calcium

Clam Chowder with Garlic Toasts

~~~~~~

My friends from New England boast about the creamy clam chowder made famous on Cape Cod and elsewhere up the coast. I love the "chowda" I sample at clam shacks from Connecticut to Maine and have come up with a version that might make me an honorary Yankee. Taste this and see if you agree.

Serves 6

For the chowder:
4 dozen littleneck clams
4 garlic cloves, minced
1 bay leaf
3 tablespoons unsalted butter
4 ounces pancetta, cut into cubes
2 celery stalks, peeled and diced
2 large shallots, diced
2 sprigs fresh thyme, leaves picked
2 tablespoons all-purpose flour
2 Yukon Gold potatoes, peeled and cubed
2 cups heavy cream
1 cup milk
¼ cup flat-leaf parsley, chopped
Freshly ground black pepper

For the garlic toasts:
1 French baguette
2 cloves garlic
¼ cup unsalted butter, softened

METHOD To prepare the chowder: Scrub the clams under cold running water to remove any dirt or sand from the shells. Place the clams, garlic, and bay leaf in a large pot and add 4 cups of water. Cover with a lid and cook for 10 to 12 minutes over medium-high heat, until all the clams have popped open (some may take longer than others to open). Lift the clams from the pot and remove the meat from the shells. Coarsely chop the clam meat and set aside. Reserve the cooking liquid from the clams.

Melt the butter in a large soup pot and add the pancetta, celery, shallots, and thyme. Cook for 5 minutes over medium-high heat or until the onion is translucent. Add the flour and stir to coat the vegetables. Add 1 cup of the reserved clam cooking liquid and whisk until there are no lumps of flour. Add the rest of the reserved cooking liquid to the pot. Add the potatoes, bring to a simmer, and cook gently for 12 to 15 minutes or until the potatoes are tender. Reduce the heat to low and add the cream and milk. Bring to a low simmer. Add the chopped littleneck clams and parsley to the pot. Season generously with freshly ground black pepper.

To prepare the garlic toasts: Preheat the oven to 425°F.

Cut the baguette in half horizontally and cut into 12 pieces. Place baguette slices on a baking sheet, cut sides up, and toast in the oven for 10 minutes or until light golden brown. Remove from the oven and rub the garlic cloves all over the toasted side of the bread. Spread the butter on the bread.

ASSEMBLY Divide the chowder between 6 serving bowls and serve with the garlic toasts alongside.

Per serving: 1,010 calories • 50 g fat • 29 g sat fat • 214 mg chol • 1497 mg sodium • 98 g carb • 6 g sugar • 5 g fiber • 45 g protein • 254 mg calcium

Orange–Poppy Seed Angel Food Cupcakes

Angel food cupcakes are a little unusual and decidedly inviting. The meringue folded into the batter makes these light and sweet, and the orange zest and poppy seeds give them unexpected yet delicious flavor and even a little crunch. Angel food cake is rarely frosted; for the cupcakes I simply top them with sweetened whipped cream.

Serves 12

For the cupcakes:
¾ cups sugar
½ cup cake flour, sifted
6 large egg whites, at room temperature
¾ teaspoon cream of tartar
⅛ teaspoon salt
Grated zest of 1 orange
1 tablespoon poppy seeds

For the frosting:
1 cup heavy cream
1 tablespoon sugar
1 teaspoon pure vanilla extract

For the garnish:
Grated zest of 1 orange

METHOD To prepare the cupcakes: Preheat the oven to 350°F.

Sift together half the sugar and the cake flour. Set aside. Using an electric mixer with the whisk attachment, whip the egg whites, 3 tablespoons of water, cream of tartar, and salt until soft peaks form. Slowly stream in the remaining sugar while continuing to whip until stiff peaks form. In three additions, fold in the sugar and flour mixture. Do not overwork. Add the orange zest and poppy seeds, stirring just to mix. Carefully but generously spoon the batter into a paper-lined 12-cup cupcake pan. Bake for 15 to 20 minutes or until the tops are golden brown and the cakes spring back when lightly touched.

Cool on a cooling rack for at least an hour before removing from the pan.

To prepare the frosting: Place the cream, sugar, and vanilla in a large mixing bowl and stir to combine. Beat until stiff peaks form. Refrigerate until ready to use.

ASSEMBLY Top the cupcakes with a dollop of the whipped cream and sprinkle with the orange zest.

Per serving: 139 calories • 8 g fat • 5 g sat fat • 27 mg chol • 60 mg sodium • 16 g carb • 10 g sugar • 1 g fiber • 3 g protein • 31 mg calcium

$\mathcal{P}$each Cobbler

~~~~~~

Peach cobbler is synonymous with summer in my book and is something my mother, Addie Mae Smith, always made us boys for a treat. I really don't recommend baking this unless the peaches are ripe and local and so juicy that they are a little tricky to slice. Buy a few extra from the farmer's market so you can eat them while waiting for the cobbler to bake.

Serves 6

For the peaches:
6 large ripe peaches, peeled, pitted, and cut into ½-inch-wide wedges
½ cup sugar
1 tablespoon cornstarch
1 teaspoon ground cinnamon
½ teaspoon ground ginger

For the topping:
1½ cups all-purpose flour
2¼ teaspoons baking powder
2½ tablespoons sugar
⅛ teaspoon salt
3 tablespoons unsalted butter, cut up and chilled
3 tablespoons vegetable shortening
½ cup buttermilk, as needed

For the garnish:
Vanilla ice cream (optional)

METHOD To prepare the peaches: Preheat the oven to 350°F.

Toss the peaches with the sugar, cornstarch, cinnamon, and ginger in a large bowl. Transfer to an 8-inch baking dish.

To prepare the topping: Combine the flour, baking powder, 1½ tablespoons of the sugar, and salt in a medium bowl. Add the cold butter and shortening and cut in with a pastry blender or a fork until the mixture looks like coarse bread crumbs. Stir in enough buttermilk to make a soft dough.

Using floured hands, pat out the dough into an 8-inch square on a floured work surface. Using a knife, cut into ¾-inch-wide ribbons. Crisscross the dough on the filling in a lattice pattern. Sprinkle the remaining 1 tablespoon of sugar over the dough.

Bake until the cobbler crust is golden brown and the filling juices are bubbling, about 45 minutes.

ASSEMBLY Spoon some of the warm cobbler into each plate and top with vanilla ice cream, if desired.

Per serving (without ice cream): 359 calories • 13 g fat • 5 g sat fat • 16 mg chol • 278 mg sodium • 60 g carb • 31 g sugar • 4 g fiber • 6 g protein • 82 mg calcium

Lemon-Yogurt Panna Cotta with Blueberries

This chilled dessert is lovely with any kind of berries, but I choose blueberries because they taste great and are also really good for you. Some nutritionists consider them a "superfood." They are high in fiber, full of vitamins C and K, and a top source of manganese. They taste really good with lemony, smooth panna cotta.

Serves 8

For the panna cotta:
¼ teaspoon canola oil
2 tablespoons fresh lemon juice
2 teaspoons unflavored gelatin
2¼ cups whole-milk Greek yogurt
1¾ cups heavy cream
¾ cup sugar

For the blueberries:
1½ cups blueberries
Grated zest of 1 lemon

METHOD To prepare the panna cotta: Lightly coat the inside of a 9-inch ceramic pie plate with the canola oil. Combine the lemon juice with 3 tablespoons water in a small bowl. Sprinkle gelatin over the mixture and stir to blend. Let stand until the gelatin softens, about 10 minutes.

Whisk the yogurt and ¾ cup of the cream in a large bowl. Combine the remaining 1 cup cream and the sugar in a small saucepan and bring to a simmer over medium heat, stirring until the sugar dissolves. Remove from the heat. Add the gelatin mixture to the hot cream mixture and whisk until the gelatin dissolves. Add the cream-gelatin mixture to the yogurt mixture and whisk to blend. Pour the panna cotta into the prepared pie plate and refrigerate until the panna cotta is set, at least 8 hours or overnight. Keep refrigerated.

Just prior to serving, run a knife around the edges of the panna cotta to loosen. Fill a large bowl with 1 inch hot water. Dip the bottom of the pie plate in the hot water for 30 seconds. Invert the panna cotta onto a large plate, and carefully lift off the pie dish.

To prepare the blueberries: Place the blueberries and ¼ cup water in a small saucepan. Cook over low heat until the blueberries are softened. Remove from the heat and add the lemon zest. Refrigerate until ready to use.

ASSEMBLY Cut the panna cotta into wedges and divide among the serving plates. Spoon the blueberries over the panna cotta.

Per serving: 331 calories • 26 g fat • 17 g sat fat • 83 mg chol • 40 mg sodium • 22 g carb • 18 g sugar • 1 g fiber • 6 g protein • 95 mg calcium

Poached Pears with Lemon Mascarpone

~~~~~~~~~~~~~~~~~~~~~~~~~~~~~~~~~~

In the fall especially, poached pears are a welcome dessert. These, flavored with a sweet, wine-y poaching liquid and topped with rich, creamy mascarpone cheese, are a lovely ending to the meal on one of those early, dark evenings when we know we're in for a long winter.

Serves 4

For the pears:
2 ripe Bosc pears, peeled, halved, and cored
2 tablespoons lemon juice
½ cup dry white wine
6 tablespoons honey
½ vanilla bean, split lengthwise

For the mascarpone:
½ cup mascarpone cheese
2 teaspoons sugar
Grated zest of 1 lemon

METHOD To prepare the pears: Toss the pears with lemon juice. In a medium saucepan, combine the wine and honey with 1 cup water. Scrape the seeds and pulp from the vanilla bean and add to the pan. Stir over medium heat until the honey is dissolved. Add the pears to the pan and cover the mixture with a round piece of parchment paper. Reduce the heat to low and simmer the pears for about 15 minutes or until tender. Remove the pears from the pan and reduce the poaching liquid to about ¾ cup. Pour the reduced poaching liquid over the pears and refrigerate until the pears are chilled.

To prepare the mascarpone: Whisk the mascarpone cheese, sugar, and lemon zest in a large bowl until smooth. Add ¼ cup of the chilled poaching syrup and whisk until soft peaks form.

ASSEMBLY Place a pear half on each plate and top with a spoonful of the lemon mascarpone.

Per serving: 420 calories • 26 g fat • 14 g sat fat • 70 mg chol • 32 mg sodium • 43 g carb • 36 g sugar • 3 g fiber • 5 g protein • 94 mg calcium

Baked Apples with Cinnamon-Oatmeal Streusel

When you don't want to make apple pie, which is high in calories and fat, bake some apples filled with a cinnamon-y streusel. They smell divine in the oven and fill the kitchen with a warm, tempting aroma—and, a little later, our stomachs with richly satisfying flavor.

Serves 4

4 large apples, such as Rome, Empire, or Honeycrisp
¼ cup packed brown sugar
¼ cup rolled oats
¼ cup unsalted butter, softened
2 tablespoons chopped dates
¼ teaspoon ground cinnamon

METHOD Preheat the oven to 425°F.

Cut the tops off the apples and core them while keeping them whole. Place the apples in an 8-inch baking dish, cored sides up.

In a small bowl, combine the brown sugar, oats, butter, dates, and cinnamon. Mix with a fork until fully incorporated. Fill each cored apple with equal amounts of the oat mixture. (Mixture will spill over the top of the apples.) Bake for 20 to 30 minutes or until the apples are tender.

ASSEMBLY Place a baked apple on each plate and serve while still warm.

Per serving: 318 calories • 12 g fat • 7 g sat fat • 31 mg chol • 5 mg sodium • 55 g carb • 42 g sugar • 6 g fiber • 2 g protein • 39 mg calcium

Strawberry Soup with Greek Frozen Yogurt

A few years ago, every restaurant I visited had fruit soup on the menu. It never really caught on as a fad, but that doesn't mean it's not 100 percent delicious! Strawberries and orange juice are a dynamite pairing, and the frozen yogurt topping is the bomb! Don't miss this one.

Serves 6

For the soup:
3 cups chopped strawberries
1 cup orange juice
2 tablespoons fresh lime juice

For the yogurt:
½ vanilla bean, cut in half lengthwise
⅔ cup sugar
2 large egg whites
3½ cups plain full-fat Greek yogurt, chilled

METHOD To prepare the soup: In a blender, combine the strawberries, orange juice, and lime juice. Process until smooth. Refrigerate the soup until chilled.

To prepare the yogurt: Scrape the seeds and pulp from the vanilla bean. In a small saucepan, combine the vanilla bean pulp and sugar with ¼ cup water and boil for 1 minute, until the sugar dissolves.

In the bowl of an electric mixer, beat the egg whites to soft peaks. Continue to beat on low while streaming in the hot sugar mixture. When all the sugar has been incorporated, turn the mixer to high and beat until the meringue is glossy and has cooled to room temperature. Fold the cold yogurt into the meringue.

Freeze the yogurt in an ice cream machine following the manufacturer's instructions. If you don't have an ice cream machine, you can pour the yogurt into a bowl and freeze. The consistency will not be a light as if prepared in an ice cream machine.

ASSEMBLY Ladle some of the chilled strawberry soup into each serving bowl and place a scoop of the frozen yogurt in the middle of the soup.

Per serving: 280 calories • 14 g fat • 11 g sat fat • 23 mg chol • 57 mg sodium • 31 g carb • 24 g sugar • 2 g fiber • 11 g protein • 136 mg calcium

~~~~~~

This soup can be frozen and shaved like a granita for a cool treat on a hot summer day. I am a big fan of perfectly ripe mangoes and they too make a great chilled soup that pairs nicely with the frozen yogurt. Simply substitute the strawberries for chopped, ripe mangoes or even papaya!

~~~~~~

Grilled Watermelon

No dessert could be easier than this one, especially when you have the grill going anyhow for an outdoor summer meal. Watermelon grilled just until grill marks appear and drizzled with lime juice is heavenly. You can serve this right away or grill it earlier in the day and refrigerate it. Don't stop with watermelon. Cantaloupe, honeydew, pineapple, mangoes, and peaches are also excellent grilled.

Serves 8

1 medium watermelon
2 tablespoons fresh lime juice

METHOD Preheat a grill to moderate flame.

Cut the watermelon into 1-inch-thick pieces. Place the watermelon on the grill and cook for 1 to 2 minutes on each side or until the watermelon gets grill marks on the flesh.

Remove the watermelon from the grill and drizzle with the lime juice. Refrigerate if desired before serving.

ASSEMBLY Arrange the watermelon on a large serving platter and enjoy.

Per serving: 170 calories • 1 g fat • 0 g sat fat • 0 mg chol • 6 mg sodium • 43 g carb • 35 g sugar • 2 g fiber • 3 g protein • 40 mg calcium

Give Yourself a Party Day!

I used to be the king of comfort and the sultan of comfort food. Those days may be over, but I will never forsake my love of both. I was raised in the deep South, where we set aside Sundays for church, feasting, and visiting. In that order. My grandmothers and mother spent a good part of every weekend preparing Sunday dinner, which more often than not included fried chicken, mac and cheese, and maybe greens. This was the one day a week we indulged in dessert—and what a treat those baked pies, cakes, and cobblers were! As indulgent as Sunday meals may have been, the greens were from our garden, the chicken from the barnyard, and the berries and fruit from a nearby patch or orchard. All fresh.

When I look back, I realize that my mother, aunts, and grandmothers were all slim and trim. They worked hard in the house and on the farm, ate wholesome food all week long, and on Sundays enjoyed the fruits of their labor. How is that for a sensible system?

I still believe in setting aside a day every week to relax and enjoy myself but not overindulge. I call this my party day. When you've worked hard all week, exercised faithfully, and watched what you put on your plate for every meal of every day, you deserve to kick back a little bit. There were innumerable times during my weight-loss journey when I nearly surrendered to a bowl of chocolate ice cream or a baked potato with sour cream. When temptation beckoned, I looked ahead. I can have that on my party day, I told myself.

Guess what! By the time the party day rolls around, I eagerly spoon some ice cream into a bowl, but I never eat as much as I might have in earlier days. Don't misunderstand: I savor every bite of chocolate, creamy macaroni and cheese, or crispy southern fried chicken, but while in the old days I might have had seconds, I no longer want more than a reasonable serving. And believe it or not, oftentimes when my party day rolls around, I find my cravings have shifted. I no longer want that peach cobbler; instead I reach for a fresh peach. Trust me, this doesn't always happen—I grew up on my mother's peach cobbler and still enjoy it to this day—but I don't need to eat it every week.

The moral of the story: as you eat less, you savor it more. Nothing wrong with that! During my journey to health and wellness, my palate and cravings shifted. I didn't crave all the sugary, fried, or high-fat foods that once soothed me. I now crave foods in their natural state with simpler preparation and cleaner flavors. Eating and cooking with whole foods has become instinctual for me, and as a result my body and mind feel much better for it. ❊

Dark Chocolate, Pumpkin Seed, and Sea Salt Bark

Chocolate bark is easy to make—just spread the melted chocolate on a baking sheet, let it cool, and then break it into pieces—but it's spectacular nonetheless. Homemade candy makes a great gift or a welcome dessert, and this is no exception. I explain how to temper the chocolate before spreading it out; doing so ensures shiny chocolate and a convincing "snap" when the chocolate is broken or bitten into.

Serves 8

1 pound bittersweet chocolate (at least 65 percent cacao), coarsely chopped
1 cup pumpkin seeds (pepitos)
1 teaspoon sea salt

METHOD Line a baking sheet with parchment paper.

To temper the chocolate, place ¾ of the chocolate in a microwave-safe bowl. Program a microwave to 50 percent power. With the bowl uncovered, heat the chocolate for 30 seconds and then stir with a rubber spatula. Repeat, heating for 30 seconds and then stirring, until almost all the chocolate in the bowl is melted, about 3 minutes total.

Using an instant-read thermometer, check the temperature of the chocolate. It should be 110°F to 115°F. If it hasn't reached desired temperature, continue to heat (in 10-second increments). Add the reserved chocolate and stir constantly until completely melted and smooth and thermometer reads 88°F to 90°F. The chocolate is now tempered.

Stir the pumpkin seeds into the chocolate.

Using an offset spatula, spread the chocolate in an even layer, about ¼ inch thick, on the parchment paper. Sprinkle the sea salt over the chocolate. Allow the bark to cool at room temperature until hard. Break into irregular pieces.

ASSEMBLY Store the bark in an airtight container at room temperature.

Per serving: 358 calories • 23 g fat • 13 g sat fat • 0 mg chol • 247 mg sodium • 41 g carb • 19 g sugar • 4 g fiber • 4 g protein • 23 mg calcium

Hibiscus-Mint Granita

~~~~~~

Granita is a light dessert, one you could enjoy any day of the week. The hibiscus flowers make it extra special and elevate the simple ice to dinner-party status. The trick to the granita's texture is to stir, or mash, it several times during freezing. This prevents it from freezing in a solid block.

Serves 4

6 dried hibiscus flowers, about ½ ounce
¾ cup sugar
Juice of 1 lime
¼ cup chopped fresh mint leaves
4 whole fresh mint leaves

METHOD Bring 2 cups water to a boil. Remove from the heat and steep the hibiscus flowers in the water for 5 to 7 minutes. Discard the hibiscus flowers. Add the sugar to the hot water and stir until melted. You may need to return it to the heat for a minute or two to dissolve the sugar. Remove from the heat and let cool to room temperature. Add the lime juice and chopped mint leaves.

Pour the liquid into a shallow bowl and place in the freezer. Freeze for 3 to 4 hours while mashing the large chunks of ice every 30 minutes or so.

ASSEMBLY Spoon the granita into chilled glasses and garnish with the whole mint leaves.

Per serving: 120 calories • 0 g fat • 0 g sat fat • 0 mg chol • 3 mg sodium • 34 g carb • 28 g sugar • 1 g fiber • 0 g protein • 26 mg calcium

A NOTE TO MY READERS

My beloveds: you have gotten this far through the book. You have laughed, you have cried, and you have seen that a 325-pound, 50-year-old chef with diabetes 2, high cholesterol, and high blood pleasure was able to change his health. The magic of this book is learning to love yourself more than the food, as my dear friend Kenny Robling told me recently. As a chef, I will always have a challenge with my weight. I love to eat. If there is one great secret, I would say that keeping supportive, positive people around you leads to success. We all feed off each other's energy, and having people around you who watch over your health is addictive. You're going to fall off and get back on the wagon of health—that's normal. But my hope is that you will become more aware of your health and realize that without it, you have nothing.

I've spent twenty years cooking for glamorous celebrities around the globe, but finally I realized that I needed to be glamorous to myself. The love of oneself leads to the better love of others. We all have the power to do great things. If you take charge of your health, you will inspire all those around you—and many more that you may not ever know. In our hungry world of lack of food to the lack of love, we realize that there is more to life.

Get comfortable with your health, as Az Ferguson says. Realize that life will be better, but also that it's going to be life changing. You're the only one who truly understands your body, and at what weight you are the happiest. Always consult with your doctor. (I don't raise a leg or an arm without asking mine.) Find that happy place and remember that a little music will help set the soundtrack of your healthy journey. "Bad Romance" by Lady Gaga keeps me churning and burning, but I also realize that to keep myself motivated, I needed to change things up. I love to run, and I've completed two marathons, but I also love boxing, and now I'm learning how to box.

You know what I want? I want to climb a mountain. Ain't no mountain high enough, and I am going to climb Mount Kilimanjaro. We all need a challenge. And remember on your journey back to health that you are human. You might fail, but if you pick yourself up and start again, you will succeed.

xoxo

ACKNOWLEDGMENTS

Great individuals showed me the road to "Healthy Comfort" but told me I had to drive to realize my dream of health and success.

My agent at CAA, Lisa Shotland, knew my health future was uncertain and searched high and low to help me find navigation. She introduced me to a beautiful man who caught my attention and my heart with "Hello, mate! We are going to find the happy!"

Az Ferguson—Aussie fitness advisor, "Health Guru" to royals, and the King of Comfort—saved and changed my life. Az, you taught me that "chef can run," and run we did, completing two marathons and two 10ks. You taught me that a forty-nine-year-old man who weighed 324 pounds, with diabetes 2, high cholesterol, and high blood pressure, could lose a large amount of weight and feel sexy again at fifty-three. My skeptical husband, Jesus Salgueiro, was also inspired by you and your work with me and has lost over thirty pounds. I am eternally grateful to you.

Jesus, you have loved me for over fourteen years and loved me when you couldn't put your arms around me. (You framed your Art and I married Jesus!) I love you and thank you for making me your husband! Our life together has never been boring, and your constant giving spirit and generosity toward others has made me a better person. I am so proud of all your work with our nonprofit, Common Threads. We founded it together at our kitchen table in 2003 and have grown it to reach thousands of children across the country!

Sari Zernich Worsham, as I ran around the world and along the beautiful shore of Lake Michigan, you watched over our company. You are the Keeper of the Art Smith Kingdom. You are not only my business partner and advisor, but also a dear friend. You have been the executive director of the Art Smith Company since we started with one restaurant, and today we have grown the company together to have five restaurants all across the country, with more to come. Your expertise as a trained chef and cookbook author made this book possible. Thank you from my healthy heart.

Bill Stankey, my book agent, and Mary Lalli of Westport Entertainment, I can't thank you enough for your many years of friendship and believing in both me and "Healthy Comfort," and that it was more than just a book.

What is a story without beautiful pictures? Stephen Hamilton's photography makes me want to eat the food right off the page! He is a dear friend and the best food photographer I know. He and his stellar team have brought my food to life in these pages. Thank you to Joanne Witherell and Paula Walters, the visionaries behind the food and prop styling, along with Lisa Kuehl and CeCe Campise.

Thanks also go to my executive editor, Nancy Hancock, and associate editor, Elsa Dixon, and their team at HarperOne for bringing the pages to life for millions to enjoy. Thank you for understanding and embracing my vision for "Healthy Comfort."

Mary Goodbody, my dear editor, we won Gourmand awards and created bestsellers; we have talked and written together for countless hours. I am grateful.

Scott Worsham, thank you for testing the recipes for the book and for being the wine and spirits advisor for the Art Smith Company. Jackie Kroon, thank you for doing the nutritional analysis of the recipes.

My dear chefs and general managers of all my restaurants across the country, I hold you all close to my heart. Chef Rey Villalobos and Mark Gallagher of TABLE Fifty-Two in Chicago; Chef Wes Morton, Chef Mike Kraus, and Patrick Chiappetta of Art and Soul, DC; Chef Timothy Magee, Chef Didier Lailheugue, and Alain Zemmour of Southern Art and Bourbon Bar, Atlanta; Chef Jeremy Bringardner of LYFE Kitchen, Palo Alto and Culver City; and Chef Travis Jones of Joanne Trattoria, New York City.

Much appreciation to Linda Novick O'Keefe, CEO of the nonprofit Common Threads, her team, and the countless volunteers for ten years of teaching thousands of children across the country. To think that with Jesus's vision and my "Barnum," together with Charles Annenberg Weingarten of The Annenberg Foundation, Thomas and Liz Pollak, and partners across the country, we will teach young America to be comfortable with their health and to make healthy food choices through the power of cooking. We have grown our mission of serving as a leader for change with regards to nutrition and health education in schools.

A journey is not possible without stopping and seeing that friends are an important part and that a positive influence is essential to success. I am grateful for Kenneth C. Robling, who kept me accountable for my health. Who taught me how to take free time instead of eating time and turning that time into cardio time. Who set that time to music that has been the soundtrack to my journey from the streets of Shanghai to the South African Savannah. My Chicago trainer, Joey Thurman, keeps me on track and moving at the gym. He introduced me to boxing, which I love and really keeps me on my toes!

I met a man in South Africa, Mike Tanchum, an entertainment lawyer who sparked my business heart. As with any heart, it has to be taught how to regulate its beat and to not allow emotion to break it. You have watched and governed over my affairs and I thank you for it.

Kevin Hauswirth, Mayor Rahm Emanuel's Media Genius Guru, you showed me how I could take my business world virtual through social networking.

Thank you, Naushab Ahmed. Man have we put on some fun events! Your humor and friendship keep me going and laughing along the way. Thank you for being my special events manager. Iris Davis, you do more than manage our home—you care for Jesus and me like family, and all our critters adore you (including our seven cats, three dogs, turtles, and fifteen fish).

Fifteen years ago, Ms. Oprah Winfrey put me on national TV and changed my life forever. Her producer Jill Barancik took my Southern Fried Chicken self and taught America to fall in love with me.

Bruce Siedel turned my humor and girth into the funny judge character on Food Network's *Iron Chef America*. Along came some mischievous elves, aka Magical Elves Productions, that took "funny" and added "sexy" and made fried chicken, Cake Gate, and the Mean Green Speedo thing something to be remembered on Bravo's *Top Chef Masters*.

Novona Cruz, you watched over my beloved boss Ms. Winfrey and are a friend to me and savior to thousands. Your new addition, as director of community affairs of the Art Smith Company, will help our company to realize more of our founding mantra, "good business doing good."

The Chef has a mother, Addie Mae Smith, who told him to keep his chin up when school bullies tried to hold him down and keeps reminding him to take care of himself. And my father, Palmer Gene Smith, who taught me to share what I love, and to my brother Gene Smith, Anise Smith, Leslie Smith, and their families, thank you for watching after the matriarch of the family and family farm.

To my friends and business partners, I am very grateful to you all!

Margie Geddes, you have believed in me all these years and have always taken my late-night calls.

Thank you Mike and Sue McCloskey for your friendship and introducing me to your delicious yogurt.

Blake Walker and Spencer Taggart, you came into my life over a blender and have given me unconditional support!

Julie and Fred Latsko, thank you for being my partners in our first restaurant. That little coach house on Elm Street has warmed countless hearts and stomachs with our Goat Cheese Drop Biscuits.

Denihan Hospitality Group and The Liaison Hotel, you helped us bring "Soul" to Capitol Hill, and shared my enthusiasm for "Fried Chicken Takes No Sides!"

Mr. John and Ellen Bortz, Pebblebrook Hotel Trust, and Intercontinental Hotel Group, you saw the vision and importance of bringing home away from home with Southern hospitality and my mother Addie Mae's Chicken and Dumpling Soup.

Joe and Cynthia Germanotta, thank you for allowing me to help you realize your dream.

Mike Roberts, Stephen Sidwell, and Mike Donahue of LYFE Kitchen, thank you for making "Unfried Chicken" the new "Fried Chicken!" We are changing the way America eats one LYFE at time. Thank you for teaching me the power of brussels sprouts!

Here is to a full life of healthy friends, healthy partners, and an abundance of comforting healthy food to share at the table with the ones you love.

xoxo
Art Smith

INDEX

~~~

Acorn Squash and Honey,
    Roasted, 182
Agave syrup, 132
Aioli, Chipotle, 132–133
Almonds, Spiced Raw, 38
Andouille sausage
    in Frogmore stew, 62
    in Jambalaya, 65–66
    White Bean Soup with, 54
Angel Food Cupcakes, Orange-
    Poppy Seed, 222–223
Antipasto, Grilled Vegetable, 34–35
Appetizers. *See* First courses;
    Snacks
Apples
    Baked, 229
    Chicken and, 76–77
Arepas, 217
Art and Soul, 15, 26, 112, 124, 128,
    170, 184
Art Start Breakfast: Steel-Cut
    Oats with Greek Yogurt and
    Blueberries, 15
Arugula
    Breakfast Sandwich, 18
    Fresh Fennel and, 72
Asparagus
    in Grilled Vegetable Antipasto,
        34–35

Halibut with Roasted
    Tomatoes and, 124–125
Slow-Cooked Farro with, 104
Avocado
    Ceviche, Shrimp and, 36
    in Crab and Endive Salad, 47
    on Fish Tacos, 133
    Guacamole, Tomatillo-, 39

Baked Apples with Cinnamon-
    Oatmeal Streusel, 229
Baked Polenta with Tomato
    Sauce and Ricotta, 102–103
Baked Sprouted Corn Chips,
    44–45
Balsamic dressing, 34–35, 74
Banana Smoothie, Kale-, 27
Banyuls vinegar, 170
Barbecue Chicken Thighs with
    Sweet Potato Salad, 150–151
Basil
    in Balsamic Dressing, 34–35
    in Chilled Pea salad, 70–71
    in Egg White Frittata, 16–17
    on Margherita Pizza, 211–212
    in polenta, 102–103, 176
    in Turkey Meat Loaf, 156–157
Basmati Rice with Spinach and
    Peas, 179–180

Beans
  Cannellini Beans and Roasted
    Fennel, 185
  Fava Bean, Radish, and Corn
    Salad, 192
  Smoky Paprika-Baked
    Garbanzo, 43
  Three-Bean Turkey Chili,
    55–56
  and Tomatoes, Green, 183
  White Bean Soup, 54
Beef
  eating, 153
  Grilled Hanger Steak, 170–171
  Short Ribs, Braised, 218–219
  Skirt Steak with Chimichurri,
    166–167
  Steak Salad, 74–75
Beets
  with Goat Cheese, 184
  Trout with Roasted Red,
    128–129
Beverages, 10, 27–29, 41, 45
Biscuits, Whole Wheat, 200–201
Black beans, 55, 98–99
Blueberry(ies)
  Lemon-Yogurt Panna Cotta
    with, 226–227
  -Peach Smoothie, 28
  Steel-Cut Oats with, 15
Blue cheese
  in Chopped Salad, 84
  –Yogurt Dressing, 76–77
Braised Beef Short Ribs with
  Carrots and Garlic-Mashed
  Potatoes, 218–219
Braised Collard Greens with
  Smoked Turkey, 194
Breads
  Arepas, 217
  Garlic Toasts, 220–221
  pizza dough, 211–212
  Whole Grain Griddle Bread,
    96–97
  Whole Wheat Biscuits, 200–201
Breakfast, 13–29
  Arepas, 217

Buckwheat Pancakes, 20–21
  Egg White Frittata, 16–17
  Oatmeal and Quinoa Granola, 26
  Sandwich, 18
  smoothies, 27–29
  Soft-Poached Egg and Root
    Vegetable Hash, 22–23
  Spinach-Feta Scramble, 24–25
  Steel-Cut Oats, 15
  Sweet Potato Waffles, 202–203
Breakfast Sandwich, 18
Bringardner, Jeremy, 27
Broccoli rabe, 34–35, 93–95,
  106–107
Broiled Salmon with Wild
  Mushrooms and Lentils,
  120–121
Broiled Sea Bass with Ginger,
  Garlic, and Carrots, 134–135
Brown rice
  Curried Pork Shoulder with,
    148–149
  Dirty Rice with Mushroom
    Bolognese, 112–113
  in Jambalaya, 65–66
  Nelson Mandela's, 179–180
Brussels sprouts
  Salad with Pine Nuts and
    Lemon, 90
  Unfried Chicken with, 160–161
Buckwheat Pancakes with
  Peaches and Greek Yogurt,
  20–21
Butter beans, 140–141
Buttermilk Dressing, 82–83
Buttermilk Fried Chicken,
  208–210

Cabbage, purple/red
  and Carrot Slaw with
    Coriander, 73
  in Fish Tacos, 132–133
Candy, chocolate bark, 234
Cannellini Beans
  and Roasted Fennel, 185
  Soup with Kale and Turkey
    Andouille Sausage, 54

in Three-Bean Turkey Chili,
  55–56
Canola oil, 87
Cantaloupe soup, 52–53
Caper(s)
  Sauce, Tomato-, 156–157
  Swordfish with, 130–131
Carrots
  with Braised Beef Short Ribs,
    218–219
  Gingered, 175
  in Purple Cabbage Slaw, 73
  Sea Bass with, 134
Catfish, Cornmeal-Crusted,
  126–127
Cauliflower
  with Pepperoncini,
    Roasted, 195
  Soup, Curried, 58–59
Celery root, 204
Ceviche, Shrimp and Avocado, 36
Charred Eggplant Tapenade, 42
Chayote Slaw, Fish Tacos with,
  132–133
Cheddar cheese, 213, 215
Cheese
  Eggplant Parmesan, 93–95
  Grilled, 213–214
  and healthy eating, 4, 5, 165, 233
  Three-Cheese Macaroni,
    215–216
  Whole Wheat Margherita
    Pizza, 211–212
  See also individual cheeses
Chicken
  and Apples with Blue Cheese–
    Yogurt Dressing, 76–77
  Barbecue Thighs, 150–151
  Buttermilk Fried, 208–210
  Garlic-Braised Thighs, 154–155
  in Jambalaya, 65–66
  Lemon-Roasted, 152–153
  and Root Vegetable Pot Pie,
    204–205
  Salad, Curried, 80–81
  Skewers with Cucumbers and
    Yogurt, 40–41

Unfried, 160–161
Chili, Three-Bean Turkey, 55–56
Chilled Peas with Heart of Palm,
  Basil, and Yogurt, 70–71
Chilled Quinoa with Smoked
  Turkey and Edamame, 78–79
Chimichurri, 166–167
Chipotle Aioli, 132–133
Chips
  Baked Sprouted Corn, 44–45
  Oven-Dried Kale, 48
Chocolate, Pumpkin Seed, and
  Sea Salt Bark, 234
Chopped Salad with Lemon
  Dressing, 84–85
Chowder, Clam, 220–221
Chowder, Miso Corn, 60
Cilantro
  in Chimichurri, 166–167
  in Fire-Roasted Tomatillo
    Salsa, 44–45
  –Pumpkin Seed Pesto, 168–169
  in Purple Cabbage and Carrot
    Slaw, 73
  in Roasted Poblano Tamales,
    100–101
  Roasted Tilapia with, 136
  in Shrimp and Avocado
    Ceviche, 36
  Sweet Corn Soup with, 57
  in Sweet Potato Salad, 150, 181
  in Tomatillo-Avocado
    Guacamole, 39
  in Watermelon and Feta
    salad, 88
Cinnamon-Oatmeal Streusel,
  Baked Apples with, 229
Clam Chowder with Garlic
  Toasts, 220–221
Cobbler, Peach, 224–225
Collard Greens with Smoked
  Turkey, Braised, 194
Coriander, Purple Cabbage and
  Carrot Slaw with, 73
Corn
  Baked Corn Chips, 44–45
  Chowder, Miso, 60

Corn (contiued)
   in Fava Bean Salad, 192
   Soup with Cilantro, 57
Cornmeal-Crusted Catfish with
   Green Tomatoes and Vidalia
   Onions, 126–127
Crab and Endive Salad, 47
Creamy Polenta with Wild
   Mushrooms, 176–177
Cucumber(s)
Chicken Skewers with, 40–41
   Edamame Hummus with, 33
   in Kale-Banana Smoothie, 27
   with Mint and Pomegranate
     Seeds, 89
   Raita, 162–163
   in Shrimp and Avocado
     Ceviche, 36
   in Yellow Tomato Gazpacho, 51
Cupcakes, Orange-Poppy Seed
   Angel Food, 222–223
Curried Cauliflower Soup, 58–59
Curried Chicken Salad with
   Whole Wheat Pita, 80–81
Curried Pork Shoulder with
   Brown Rice and Mustard
   Greens, 148–149
Curried Quinoa, 178–179
Custard, Spinach, 187

Dalai Lama, 108
Dark Chocolate, Pumpkin Seed,
   and Sea Salt Bark, 234
Desserts
   Baked Apples, 229
   Grilled Watermelon, 232
   Hibiscus-Mint Granita, 235
   Lemon-Yogurt Panna Cotta,
     226–227
   Orange–Poppy Seed Angel
     Food Cupcakes, 222–223
   Peach Cobbler, 224–225
   Poached Pears, 228
   Strawberry Soup, 230–231
Dill Dressing, 128–129
Dips
   Edamame Hummus, 33

Fire-Roasted Tomatillo Salsa,
   44–45
   Tomatillo-Avocado
     Guacamole, 39
Dirty Rice with Mushroom
   Bolognese, 112–113
Dressings
   balsamic, 34–35, 74
   Blue Cheese–Yogurt, 76–77
   Buttermilk, 82–83
   Dill, 128–129
   lemon, 72, 84–85
Drinks, 10, 27–29, 41, 45

Edamame
   in Chilled Quinoa salad, 78–79
   Hummus with Cucumber
     Slices, 33
Eggplant
   Parmesan with Garlic Rapini,
     93–95
   Tapenade, Charred, 42
Egg(s)
   Breakfast Sandwich, 18
   in Chopped Salad, 84
   on Creamy Polenta, 177
   over Oatmeal Risotto with
     Shrimp, 138–139
   Soft-Poached, 22–23
   Spinach-Feta Scramble,
     24–25
   White Frittata with Roasted
     Mushrooms, Goat Cheese,
     and Basil, 16–17
Endive Salad, Crab and, 47
Escarole Soup, Lentil and, 63–64
Exercise
   importance of, 7, 11, 23
   running, 9–10, 56
   during travel, 37

Farmer cheese, 100–101
Farro with Asparagus and
   Pecorino Cheese, 104
Fats, 6, 38, 87, 159
Fava Bean, Radish, and Corn
   Salad, 192

Fennel
 and Arugula with Meyer
  Lemon Dressing, 72
 Cannellini Beans and, 185
Ferguson, Aaron (Az), 3, 7, 9–12,
 19, 56
Feta cheese
 Spinach-Feta Scramble, 24–25
 Watermelon and, 88
Field Pea and Hominy Succotash,
 190–191
Fire-Roasted Tomatillo Salsa and
 Baked Sprouted Corn Chips,
 44–45
First courses
 Charred Eggplant
  Tapenade, 42
 Chicken Skewers, 40–41
 Grilled Shisho Peppers, 46
 Grilled Vegetable Antipasto,
  34–35
 Shrimp and Avocado
  Ceviche, 36
 See also Salads; Soups
Fish main courses
 Broiled Salmon, 120–121
 Broiled Sea Bass, 134–135
 Cornmeal-Crusted Catfish,
  126–127
 Fish Tacos, 132–133
 Glazed Salmon, 122–123
 Halibut, 124–125
 Roasted Tilapia, 136–137
 Swordfish, 130–131
 Trout, 128–129
Fish Tacos with Chayote Slaw
 and Chipotle Aioli, 132–133
Fitzsimons, Kevin, 108
Fontina cheese, 206–207, 215
Fresh Fennel and Arugula with
 Meyer Lemon Dressing, 72
Frittata
 Egg White, 16–17
 spinach-feta, 25
Frogmore Stew, 62
Frozen Yogurt, Strawberry Soup
 with Greek, 230–231

Fruit
 Baked Apples, 229
 Chicken and Apples, 76–77
 daily servings, 110–111
 Grilled Watermelon, 232
 Lemon-Yogurt Panna Cotta
  with Blueberries, 226–227
 Melon Soup, 52–53
 Peach Cobbler, 224–225
 Poached Pears, 228
 shakes, 41
 Smoothies, 27–29
 Strawberry Soup, 230–231
 Watermelon and Feta, 88

Garbanzo Beans, Smoky Paprika-
 Baked, 43
Garden Greens with Buttermilk
 Dressing, 82–83
Garlic
 -Braised Chicken Thighs with
  Quinoa, 154–155
 Broiled Sea Bass with,
  134–135
 -Mashed Potatoes, 218–219
 Rapini, Eggplant Parmesan
  with, 93–95
 Toasts, 220–221
Gazpacho, Yellow Tomato, 51
Germanotta, Cynthia and
 Joseph, 206
Ginger
 in Roasted Sweet Potato
  soup, 61
 Sea Bass with, 134
 Steamed Mussels with, 142
Gingered Carrots, 175
Goat cheese, 25
 in Egg White Frittata, 16–17
Griddle Bread with, 96–97
Grilled Shisho Peppers Stuffed
 with, 46
 Pickled Red Beets with, 184
 in Potato Tart, 108–109
Granita, Hibiscus-Mint, 235
Granola, Oatmeal and
 Quinoa, 26

Greek Frozen Yogurt, Strawberry Soup with, 230–231
Greek yogurt
    Blueberry-Peach Smoothie, 28
    Blue Cheese–Yogurt Dressing, 76–77
    Buckwheat Pancakes with, 20–21
    Chicken Skewers with Cucumbers and, 40–41
    in Chilled Peas salad, 70–71
    in Chipotle Aioli, 132–133
    in Cucumber Raita, 162–163
    in Lemon-Yogurt Panna Cotta, 226–227
    Mango, Mint, and Pineapple Smoothie, 29
    Steel-Cut Oats with Blueberries and, 15
Green Beans and Tomatoes, 183
Green Tomatoes and Vidalia Onions, Cornmeal-Crusted Catfish with, 126–127
Griddle Bread with Goat Cheese, Whole Grain, 96–97
Grilled Cheese, 213–214
Grilled Flank Steak Salad with Red Onions, Tomatoes, and Spinach, 74–75
Grilled Hanger Steak with Slow-Roasted Tomatoes and Watercress, 170–171
Grilled Radicchio, 193
Grilled Shisho Peppers Stuffed with Goat Cheese, 46
Grilled Watermelon, 232
Guacamole, Tomatillo-Avocado, 39

Halibut with Roasted Tomatoes and Asparagus, 124–125
Hash, Root Vegetable, 22–23
Healthy eating
    and balance, 19
    carbohydrates, 59, 191
    eating out, 164–165
    on fats, 6, 38, 87, 159
    food choices, 4–5

food shopping, 105
    overview of, 1–7, 10–11
    while traveling, 37
    whole foods, 4, 59, 105, 191
    whole foods for, 4, 59
Healthy lifestyle
    controlling diabetes, 2–3, 10–11
    vs. sedentary, 71
    support systems, xiv, 79
Hearts of palm salad, 70–71
Herb-and-Mustard-Crusted Pork Tenderloin with Roasted Peaches, 158–159
Hibiscus-Mint Granita, 235
Hominy
    Shrimp and, 140–141
    Succotash, Field Pea and, 190–191
Honey
    Roasted Acorn Squash and, 182
    Whole Wheat Biscuits with Crushed Strawberries and, 200–201
Hummus with Cucumber Slices, Edamame, 33

Iron Chef, 143

Jambalaya, 65–66
Joanne Trattoria, 206–207
Jones, Quincy, 134

Kalamata olives, 130–131
Kale
    -Banana Smoothie, 27
    Chips, Oven-Dried, 48
    in Feta Scramble, 24–25
    -Stuffed Turkey Meat Loaf with Tomato-Caper Sauce, 156–157
    and Summer Squash salad, 86
    White Bean Soup with, 54
Kefir
    Blueberry-Peach Smoothie, 28
    Mango, Mint, and Pineapple Smoothie, 29

Kidney beans, 55
King, Gayle, 23

Lady Gaga, 206, 208
Lamb Kabobs with Cucumber
    Raita, 162–163
Lasagna, Zucchini, 206–207
Leeks, Roasted, 186
Lemon
    Dressing, 84–85
    Mascarpone, 228
    Ricotta, Sweet Potato Waffles
        with, 202–203
    -Roasted Chicken with Banana
        Peppers, 152–153
    Roasted Tilapia with, 136
    Shaved Brussels Sprout Salad
        with Pine Nuts and, 90
    Spinach-Feta Scramble with,
        24–25
    Sugar Snap Peas with, 188
    -Yogurt Panna Cotta with
        Blueberries, 226–227
Lemon Thyme, Potato Tart with
    Mustard Greens and, 108–109
Lentil(s)
    Broiled Salmon with Wild
        Mushrooms and, 120–121
    and Escarole Soup with
        Manchego Cheese, 63–64
Lima beans, 140–141
Lime
    and Mint Scallops with Red
        Onion, 118–119
    Watermelon and Feta with, 88
LYFE Kitchen, 15, 16, 18, 27, 33,
    92, 93, 132, 138, 160

Macaroni, Three-Cheese, 215–216
Mahi mahi, 132–133
Manchego Cheese, Lentil and
    Escarole Soup with, 63–64
Mandela, Nelson, 179
Mango
    frozen yogurt soup, 231
    Mint, and Pineapple
        Smoothie, 29

Masa harina, 100
Masarepa cornmeal, 217
Mascarpone, Lemon, 228
Meat Loaf, Kale-Stuffed Turkey,
    156–157
Meat main courses. See individual
    meats
Melon Soup with Grilled Shrimp,
    52–53
Meyer Lemon Dressing, 72
Mint
    Cucumbers with, 89
    Granita, Hibiscus-, 235
    Mango, and Pineapple
        Smoothie, 29
    Scallops with Red Onion, Lime
        and, 118–119
Mirliton, 132
Miso Corn Chowder, 60
Mornay cheese sauce, 215
Mushroom(s)
    Bolognese, 112–113
    Broiled Salmon with Wild,
        120–121
    Creamy Polenta with Wild,
        176–177
    in Egg White Frittata, 16–17
    in Shirataki Noodles Stir-Fry,
        106–107
Mussels with Ginger and Thai
    Red Chilies, Steamed, 142
Mustard greens
    Curried Pork Shoulder with,
        148–149
    in Feta Scramble, 25
    Potato Tart with, 108–109

Nelson Mandela's Brown Basmati
    Rice with Spinach and Peas,
    179–180
Nutritional yeast, 48

Oatmeal
    Art Start Breakfast, 15
    benefits of, 5, 10, 13, 17
    Cinnamon-Oatmeal Streusel,
        Baked Apples with, 229

Oatmeal (continued)
   and Quinoa Granola, 26
   Risotto with Shrimp and
      Sweet Peas, 138–139
Obama, Barack, 23, 122–123
Obama, Michelle, 122
Oils, 87
Olives, Swordfish with, 130–131
Onions
   Grilled Flank Steak Salad with
      Red, 74–75
   Lime and Mint Scallops with
      Red, 118–119
   Vidalia, Cornmeal-Crusted
      Catfish with, 126–127
Orange–Poppy Seed Angel Food
   Cupcakes, 222–223
Oranges, 72
Ornish, Dean, 134
Oven-Dried Kale Chips, 48
Oz, Mehmet, 211

Pancakes, Buckwheat, 20–21
Panna Cotta with Blueberries,
   Lemon-Yogurt, 226–227
Paprika-Baked Garbanzo Beans,
   Smoky, 43
Parmesan cheese
   in Creamy Polenta, 176–177
   in Dirty Rice, 112–113
   in Eggplant Parmesan, 93–95
   on Margherita Pizza, 211–212
   in Oatmeal Risotto, 138–139
   Zucchini Lasagna, 206–207
Parsnips, 204–205
Pasta dishes
   Three-Cheese Macaroni,
      215–216
   Whole Wheat Penne,
      Swordfish with, 130–131
   Zucchini Lasagna, 206–207
Pasta sauce, 93–94
Pea and Hominy Succotash, Field,
   190–191
Peach(es)
   Blueberry-Peach Smoothie, 28

Buckwheat Pancakes with,
   20–21
Cobbler, 224–225
Pork Tenderloin with Roasted,
   158–159
Pears with Lemon Mascarpone,
   Poached, 228
Peas
   Brown Basmati Rice with,
      179–180
   in Chicken and Root Vegetable
      Pot Pie, 204–205
   with Heart of Palm, 70–71
   with Lemon, 188
   in Lime and Mint Scallops,
      118–119
   Steel-Cut Oatmeal Risotto
      with Shrimp and, 138–139
Pecorino Romano cheese
   in Kale-Stuffed Turkey Meat
      Loaf, 156–157
   Slow-Cooked Farro with, 104
Penne, 130–131
Pepitos, 86, 168–169
Pepperoncini, Roasted
   Cauliflower with, 195
Peppers
   in Garlic-Braised Chicken,
      154–155
   Grilled Shisho, 46
   in Grilled Vegetable Antipasto,
      34–35
   Lemon-Roasted Chicken with,
      152–153
   Poblano Tamales, 100–101
   serrano in watermelon salad, 88
Pesto, Cilantro–Pumpkin Seed,
   168–169
Phyllo dough, whole wheat,
   108–109
Pickled Red Beets with Goat
   Cheese, 184
Pineapple Smoothie, Mango,
   Mint, and, 29
Pine Nuts, Shaved Brussels
   Sprout Salad with, 90

Pizza, Whole Wheat Margherita, 211–212
Poached Pears with Lemon Mascarpone, 228
Poblano Tamales, Roasted, 100–101
Poitier, Sidney, 130
Polenta
    with Tomato Sauce and Ricotta, Baked, 102–103
    with Wild Mushrooms, Creamy, 176–177
Pomegranate Seeds, Cucumber with Mint and, 89
Poppy Seed Angel Food Cupcakes, Orange-, 222–223
Pork
    Chops with Cilantro–Pumpkin Seed Pesto, 168–169
    with Cilantro–Pumpkin Seed Pesto, 168–169
    Curried, 148–149
    Tenderloin, Herb-and-Mustard-Crusted, 158–159
Potato(es)
    in Chicken and Root Vegetable Pot Pie, 204–205
    Garlic-Mashed, 218–219
    Roasted Fingerling, 166–167
    Tart with Mustard Greens and Lemon Thyme, 108–109
    in Vegetable Shepherd's Pie, 98–99
Pot Pie, Chicken and Root Vegetable, 204–205
Poultry. See Chicken; Turkey
President Barack Obama's Favorite Glazed Salmon, 122–123
Protein, 145–146, 153
Pumpkin Seed(s)
Pesto, Cilantro-, 168–169
    and Sea Salt Bark, Dark Chocolate, 234
Purple Cabbage and Carrot Slaw with Coriander, 73

Queso fresco, 100–101
Quinoa
    Chilled, with Smoked Turkey and Edamame, 78–79
    Curried, 178–179
    Garlic-Braised Chicken Thighs with, 154–155
    Granola, Oatmeal and, 26
    with Lamb Kabobs, 162–163

Radicchio
    in Chopped Salad, 84
    Grilled, 193
Radishes
    in Fava Bean Salad, 192
    on Trout with Roasted Red Beets, 128–129
Raita, 162–163
Raizer, Jeffrey, 56
Rapini
    in Eggplant Parmesan, 93–95
    in Grilled Vegetable Antipasto, 34–35
    in Shirataki Noodles Stir-Fry, 106–107
Red Beets with Goat Cheese, Pickled, 184
Red cabbage
    in Fish Tacos, 132–133
Red onion(s)
    Grilled Flank Steak Salad with, 74–75
    Lime and Mint Scallops with, 118–119
Rice, brown. See Brown rice
Ricotta cheese
    in Baked Polenta, 102–103
    in Eggplant Parmesan, 93–95
    Lemon, 202–203
    in Zucchini Lasagna, 206–207
Ricotta salata, 86
Risotto with Shrimp and Sweet Peas, 138–139
Roasted Acorn Squash and Honey, 182

Roasted Cauliflower with
Pepperoncini, 195
Roasted Leeks, 186
Roasted Poblano Tamales,
100–101
Roasted Sweet Potato and Ginger
Soup, 61
Roasted Tilapia with Lemon and
Cilantro, 136–137
Robling, Kenneth, 12, 23, 79, 211
Romano cheese, 104, 156–157
Ronnen, Tal, 33, 92, 108
Root Vegetable Hash, 22–23
Root Vegetable Pot Pie, 204–205
Rutabagas, 22–23

Salads, 70–90
about, 5, 67–68, 111
Chicken and Apples, 76–77
Chilled Peas with Heart of
Palm, 70–71
Chilled Quinoa with Turkey
and Edamame, 78–79
Chopped, 84–85
Crab and Endive, 47
Cucumber, 89
Curried Chicken, 80–81
Fava Bean, Radish, and Corn, 192
Fresh Fennel and Arugula, 72
Garden Greens, 82–83
Grilled Flank Steak, 74–75
Purple Cabbage and Carrot
Slaw, 73
Shaved Brussels Sprout with
Pine Nuts, 90
Shrimp and Avocado
Ceviche, 36
Sweet Potato, 150–151, 181
tzatziki, 40–41
Warm Kale and Summer
Squash, 86
Watermelon and Feta, 88
See also Dressings
Salgueiro, Jesus, 217
Salmon
President Barack Obama's
Favorite Glazed, 122–123

with Wild Mushrooms and
Lentils, Broiled, 120–121
Salsa, Fire-Roasted Tomatillo,
44–45
Sandwich(es)
Breakfast, 18
Curried Chicken Salad, 80–81
Grilled Cheese, 213–214
tips on, 111
Sauces
barbecue, 150–151
cheese, 206–207
chimichurri, 166–167
Chipotle Aioli, 132–133
Cilantro–Pumpkin Seed Pesto,
168–169
Cucumber Raita, 162–163
Mornay cheese, 215
tomato, 93–95, 102–103, 130–
131, 156–157
Sausage, turkey. See Turkey
sausage
Scallops with Red Onion, Lime
and Mint, 118–119
Sea Bass with Ginger, Garlic, and
Carrots, 134–135
Seafood main courses
Lime and Mint Scallops,
118–119
Oatmeal Risotto with Shrimp,
138–139
Shrimp and Hominy, 140–141
Steamed Mussels, 142
Sea Salt Bark, Dark Chocolate,
Pumpkin Seed, and, 234
Serrano Chili Peppers,
Watermelon and Feta with, 88
Shaved Brussels Sprout Salad
with Pine Nuts and Lemon, 90
Shepherd's Pie, Vegetable, 98–99
Shiitake mushrooms, 106, 176
Shirataki Noodles Stir-Fry,
106–107
Shotland, Lisa, 9
Shrimp
and Avocado Ceviche, 36
and Hominy, 140–141

in Jambalaya, 65–66
    Melon Soup with Grilled, 52–53
    Oatmeal Risotto with, 138–139
Skirt Steak with Chimichurri and
    Roasted Fingerling Potatoes,
    166–167
Slaw, Purple Cabbage and
    Carrot, 73
Slow-Cooked Farro with
    Asparagus and Pecorino
    Cheese, 104
Slow-Roasted Tomatoes, 189
Smoky Paprika-Baked Garbanzo
    Beans, 43
Smoothies
    Blueberry-Peach, 28
    Kale-Banana, 27
    Mango, Mint, and Pineapple, 29
Snacks
    about, 31–32, 41
    Charred Eggplant Tapenade, 42
    Edamame Hummus, 33
    Fire-Roasted Tomatillo Salsa,
    44–45
    Grilled Vegetable Antipasto,
    34–35
    Oven-Dried Kale Chips, 48
    Smoky Paprika-Baked
    Garbanzo Beans, 43
    Spiced Raw Almonds, 38
    Tomatillo-Avocado
    Guacamole, 39
Soft-Poached Egg and Root
    Vegetable Hash, 22–23
Soups, 49–66
    about, 49–50
    chilled, 51–53, 230–231
    Clam Chowder, 220–221
    Curried Cauliflower, 58–59
    Lentil and Escarole, 63–64
    Melon with Grilled Shrimp,
    52–53
    Miso Corn Chowder, 60
    Roasted Sweet Potato and
    Ginger, 61
    Strawberry, 230–231
    Sweet Corn with Cilantro, 57

Tomato, 213–214
    White Bean with Kale and
    Sausage, 54
    Yellow Tomato Gazpacho, 51
    See also Stews
Southern Art, 84, 140, 190
Soybeans, 78–79
Spiced Raw Almonds, 38
Spinach
    Brown Basmati Rice with,
    179–180
    Custard, 187
    -Feta Scramble with Lemon,
    24–25
    in Grilled Flank Steak Salad,
    74–75
Squash
    in Grilled Vegetable Antipasto,
    34–35
    Kale and Summer, 86
    Roasted Acorn, 182
    Zucchini Lasagna, 206–207
Steak Salad, 74–75
Steamed Mussels with Ginger
    and Thai Red Chilies, 142
Steel-Cut Oatmeal Risotto with
    Shrimp and Sweet Peas,
    138–139
Steel-Cut Oats with Greek Yogurt
    and Blueberries, 15
Stews
    Curried Pork Shoulder, 148–149
    Frogmore, 62
    Jambalaya, 65–66
    Three-Bean Turkey Chili,
    55–56
Stir-Fry, Shirataki Noodles,
    106–107
Strawberries, Whole Wheat
    Biscuits with Crushed,
    200–201
Strawberry Soup with Greek
    Frozen Yogurt, 230–231
Succotash, Field Pea and Hominy,
    190–191
Sugar, 6, 13–14, 214
Sugar Snap Peas with Lemon, 188

Sunflower oil, 87
Sweet Corn Soup with
    Cilantro, 57
Sweet potato(es)
    in Chicken and Root Vegetable
        Pot Pie, 204–205
    and Ginger Soup, Roasted, 61
    in Root Vegetable Hash, 22–23
    in salad, 150–151, 181
    Waffles with Lemon Ricotta,
        202–203
Sweet Potato Salad with Cumin
    and Cilantro, 181
Swordfish with Capers, Olives,
    Tomato Sauce, and Whole
    Wheat Penne, 130–131

TABLE Fifty-Two, 62, 194, 195,
    208, 215
Tacos with Chayote Slaw, Fish,
    132–133
Tamales, Roasted Poblano,
    100–101
Tapenade, Charred Eggplant, 42
Thai Red Chilies, Steamed
    Mussels with, 142
Three-Bean Turkey Chili, 55–56
Three-Cheese Macaroni, 215–216
Thurman, Joey, 12
Tilapia with Lemon and Cilantro,
    Roasted, 136–137
Togarashi spice, 52
Tomatillo
    -Avocado Guacamole, 39
    Salsa, Fire-Roasted, 44–45
Tomato(es)
    and Asparagus, Halibut with
        Roasted, 124–125
    Cornmeal-Crusted Catfish
        with Green, 126–127
    Green Beans and, 183
    in Grilled Flank Steak Salad,
        74–75
    Slow-Roasted, 170–171, 189
    Soup and Grilled Cheese,
        213–214
    Yellow Tomato Gazpacho, 51

Tomato sauce
    Baked Polenta with, 102–103
    with capers, 156–157
    for Eggplant Parmesan, 93–95
    Swordfish with, 130–131
Top Chef, 1, 108, 143
Tortilla chips, 44
Trout with Roasted Red Beets,
    Radishes, and Dill Dressing,
    128–129
Turkey
    Braised Collard Greens with
        Smoked, 194
    Chili, Three-Bean, 55–56
    Chilled Quinoa with Smoked,
        78–79
    Meat Loaf, Kale-Stuffed,
        156–157
Turkey sausage
    Breakfast Sandwich, 18
    in Frogmore Stew, 62
    in Jambalaya, 65–66
    White Bean Soup with
        Kale, 54
Turnips, 22–23
Tzatziki, 40–41

Unfried Chicken with Roasted
    Brussels Sprouts, 160–161

Vegetables, 173–195
    adding to soup, 49–50
    daily servings, 110–111
    Grilled Vegetable Antipasto,
        34–35
    Root Vegetable Hash, 22–23
    Root Vegetable Pot Pie,
        Chicken and, 204–205
    See also individual vegetables
Vegetable Shepherd's Pie, 98–99
Vegetarian main courses, 91–113
    Baked Polenta, 102–103
    Dirty Rice with Mushroom
        Bolognese, 112–113
    Eggplant Parmesan, 93–95
    Potato Tart with Mustard
        Greens, 108–109

Roasted Poblano Tamales, 100–101

Shirataki Noodles Stir-Fry, 106–107

Slow-Cooked Farro with Asparagus, 104

Vegetable Shepherd's Pie, 98–99
  Whole Grain Griddle Bread with Goat Cheese, 96–97

Vidalia Onions, Cornmeal-Crusted Catfish with, 126–127

Villalobos, Rey, 108, 208

Waffles with Lemon Ricotta, Sweet Potato, 202–203

Warm Kale and Summer Squash with Ricotta Salata, 86

Watercress, 170–171

Watermelon
  and Feta with Lime and Serrano Chili Peppers, 88
  Grilled, 232

Wheat berries, 104

White Bean Soup with Kale and Turkey Andouille Sausage, 54

Whole Grain Griddle Bread with Goat Cheese, 96–97

Whole Wheat Biscuits with Crushed Strawberries and Honey, 200–201

Whole Wheat Margherita Pizza, 211–212

Whole Wheat Penne, Swordfish with, 130–131

Whole wheat phyllo dough, 108–109

Winfrey, Oprah, 3, 23, 122, 130, 134, 143, 160, 179, 208

Wong, Alan, 122

Yam flour noodles, 106–107

Yellow Tomato Gazpacho, 51

Yogurt, Greek. *See* Greek yogurt

Zucchini
  Grilled Vegetable Antipasto, 34–35
  Lasagna from Joanne Trattoria, 206–207
  in Lemon-Roasted Chicken, 152–153

SCAN THIS CODE

WITH YOUR SMARTPHONE TO BE LINKED TO
THE BONUS MATERIALS FOR

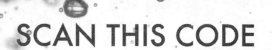

ART SMITH'S HEALTHY COMFORT

on the Elixir mobile website,
where you can also find information about other
healthy living books and related materials.

YOU CAN ALSO TEXT

ARTSMITH to READIT (732348)

to be sent a link to the Elixir mobile website.

 Facebook.com/elixirliving   Twitter.com/elixirliving   www.elixirliving.com